Guide to the Guidelines

Volume 3

Pancreaticobiliary and Liver Diseases

A vignette-based journey through the ACG clinical practice guidelines

Brennan Spiegel, MD, MSHS, FACG
and
Hetal A. Karsan, MD, FACG

Published by The American College of Gastroenterolgy
American College of Gastroenterology
11333 Woodglen Drive, Suite 100
North Bethesda, MD 20852, USA

This book is intended as an educational resource for healthcare professionals and should not replace individual clinical judgment. The authors and the American College of Gastroenterology (ACG) make no guarantees regarding the accuracy or completeness of the information presented and assume no liability for any errors, omissions, or consequences arising from the application of the content. Clinicians are encouraged to consult relevant guidelines directly and use their discretion in applying information from this book to patient care.

ISBN: 9798218824860

Contents

Preface
Know Your Guidelines!

"What do the ACG guidelines say?"

If you're a practicing gastroenterologist or hepatologist, then that's an excellent question. It's a question you probably ask yourself every day you are in clinic or at the hospital. It's a question that determines how best to diagnose, treat, and deliver the highest quality care for patients with digestive diseases. The bottom line is this: you really must know the guidelines!

Of course, the best way to know the guidelines is to read them. As of this writing, the American College of Gastroenterology (ACG) has published over 70 guidelines covering diseases of the esophagus, to disorders of the anorectum, to, well, just about everywhere else between the poles of the alimentary canal. These documents are pure gold. They lay out, in evidence-based splendor, the key recommendations that govern clinical practice in our field. They are required reading.

But let's be fair about something. Reading through 70+ guidelines encompassing well over 4,000 pages of text and drawing from over 10,000 citations is not easy sledding. By the time you reach the end of the guidelines, you probably need to start over because (a) you forgot some things; (b) the guidelines are periodically revised; and (c) new guidelines are constantly in the works.

That's why we wrote this book. As a former Editor-in-Chief of *The American Journal of Gastroenterology* (B.S.) and former editor of the Journal's "Red Section" (H.K.), we have observed a strong desire among clinicians to learn the guidelines in efficient, accessible, and fun ways. We discovered that our most popular Journal podcasts are those about the ACG guidelines and the most successful Red Section columns were authored by senior clinicians who interpreted the guidelines through an expert lens shaped by years of practice.

We got to thinking—wouldn't it be handy to have a "guide to the guidelines" that digested (pun intended) the 4,000 pages of ACG documents into a concise, entertaining, and useful review of the most salient pearls and insights? We imagined a resource that would reflect the accessible style of our AJG podcasts with the pragmatic lessons in the most popular Red Section columns. Also, because clinicians learn by example, we figured that a vignette-based journey through the guidelines would bring the ACG material to life in ways that a typical textbook might fall short (peeps love to learn from vignettes). That led to the book you are reading now.

Here's how we structured *Guide to the Guidelines*, which we call G2G for short: We mapped each of the ACG guidelines into one of three major topics. Each topic composes 1 of 3 volumes for the G2G series. You are now holding Volume 3, titled *Pancreaticobiliary and Liver*. In Chapter One, "Don't Mess with the Pancreas," we summarize all the guidelines on acute pancreatitis, chronic pancreatitis, and pancreatic cysts. Chapter Two, "Bile and Brimstone," reviews the guidelines on various biliary disorders, including primary sclerosing cholangitis (PSC) and management of bile duct strictures. Finally, in Chapter Three, "Liver Me Timbers!," we cover the many and splendorous ACG guidelines on liver diseases, including alcohol-associated liver disease and malnutrition, liver test interpretation, acute liver failure, drug-induced liver injury, acute-on-chronic liver failure, focal liver lesions, liver disease and pregnancy, hereditary hemochromatosis, and disorders of the hepatic and mesenteric circulation. That's right, it's liver, liver and more liver! That's right, it's liver, liver, and more liver!

If you haven't already seen Volume 1, entitled *Bread and Butter GI* (also called the "Red Book") or Volume 2, entitled *GI Infections, Inflammation, and Bleeding* (the "Blue Book"), go check them out! And now with this book, which we'll call the "Green Book," we have completed the full G2G trilogy. Gift it to your kids for the holidays!

Each G2G chapter includes carefully selected vignettes designed to illustrate key concepts from the guidelines, followed by a conversation-style discussion written to keep you awake and alert. As you read these discussions, you'll notice that we highlight specific points along the margin that we think are especially noteworthy. Then, following each chapter, we provide multiple choice questions to test your knowledge of the material. We prepared questions that highlight information we believe is most vital to ensure high quality care, as judged by our nearly 50 years (and counting...) of combined experience managing GI and liver patients in both academic and private practice settings (yikes, we're getting old). We also worked with the authors of each ACG guideline to ensure that our treatment of their document is accurate and thank them all for their time and commitment to this ACG project. We hope you find the discussions and questions to be both enjoyable and useful.

This is an example of how we highlight points in the margin

Because the ACG guidelines are constantly revised and updated, the book you are now reading will eventually become outdated. In fact, it might already be outdated! That's the nature of guidelines. It's important to keep up with the latest recommendations because they often change meaningfully as scientific evidence emerges. We will continue to update this book to ensure it remains modern and accurate. Life is a work in progress.

We hope you enjoy reading the G2G trilogy as much as we enjoyed writing all of these books. If nothing else, preparing this comprehensive resource in partnership with the ACG helped us learn the guidelines and we trust it will help you too.

Brennan Spiegel, MD, MSHS, FACG
Professor of Medicine and Public Health
Gourrich Chair in Digital Health Ethics
Director of Health Services Research, Cedars-Sinai
Director, Cedars-Sinai Master's Degree Program in Health Delivery Science

Hetal A. Karsan, MD, FACG
Chair of Credentials Committee, ACG
International Governor, ACG
Chair of Medical Education, United Digestive
Adjunct Professor of Medicine, Emory University

Chapter One

Don't Mess with the Pancreas

The Enzyme Bug that Bites Back

If there's one organ that teaches you humility on call, it's the pancreas. What might start as a case of mere abdominal pain can quickly unravel into hours of fluids, labs, repeat imaging, and increasingly urgent consults. This is not a gland to take lightly. Whether it's acutely inflamed, chronically scarred, or hiding something cystic, the pancreas makes you earn your keep. Every surgeon knows this well: don't mess with the pancreas!

In this chapter, we walk through the ACG's latest guidance on acute pancreatitis, chronic pancreatitis, and pancreatic cysts. From early diagnosis (spoiler: lipase is more helpful than amylase) to when to scan, when to scope, and when to leave things alone, we've got you covered. This stuff is straight-up, high-yield material for everyday clinical practice. We'll cover the step-up strategy for infected necrosis, how to decode pain in chronic pancreatitis (and why it's not always about the enzymes), and when to start worrying about that "simple" cyst in the tail that keeps showing up on follow-up imaging.

We're sticking to the guidelines—2024 for acute pancreatitis, 2020 for chronic, and yes, the 2018 cyst guideline still holds up for now while the new ones are being finished. These are high-yield, clinic-ready, guidelines that you're bound to use the next time you are on call.

And of course, once you're done with the chapter, there's a quiz at the end to see if you're still standing—or if the pancreas got the last laugh.

Case 1.1: A Pain in the Back

A 36-year-old woman presents to the emergency department (ED) with upper abdominal pain that began the previous evening. The pain is severe, centered in the epigastrium, and radiates to her back. It is constant and associated with nausea and vomiting. She does not report fevers, recent infections, or trauma. Her past medical history includes hyperlipidemia, and she drinks alcohol socially. The night prior, she had a large meal and several alcoholic beverages.

On exam, she is afebrile, normotensive, and mildly tachycardic. Abdominal exam reveals tenderness to palpation in the epigastrium without rebound or guarding. Laboratory testing shows: white blood cell (WBC): 12.4 K/µL; serum lipase: 942 U/L (upper limit normal [ULN]: 60 U/L); amylase: 283 U/L; transaminases are within normal limits; triglycerides are pending.

Abdominal ultrasound reveals cholelithiasis with no biliary ductal dilation. The pancreas is not well-visualized due to overlying bowel gas.

The ED team is considering a diagnosis of acute pancreatitis and requests input on the next steps, including whether additional imaging is needed.

Know your guidelines!

1. Does this patient meet criteria for a diagnosis of acute pancreatitis?
2. When is imaging indicated in suspected acute pancreatitis?
3. Is it necessary for both amylase and lipase to be elevated?
4. Could this patient have acute pancreatitis with a normal lipase level?

Case 1.1: What do the guidelines say?

Source: ACG 2024 Acute Pancreatitis Guidelines[1]

The ACG's 2024 guideline on acute pancreatitis (AP) is super clear on this point: AP is overwhelmingly a **clinical** diagnosis, and our patient already checks the requisite boxes. The guideline asks us to confirm any 2 of the following 3 elements shown in **Table 1.1**.

Table 1.1. *The "2-of-3" rule for diagnosing AP. The ACG guideline reminds us that AP is a clinical diagnosis requiring any 2 of the 3 diagnostic elements.*

Diagnostic element	Practical notes
Typical acute pancreatitis pain—steady, severe, epigastric or left upper quadrant, often boring to the back	Colicky lower abdomen discomfort or fleeting cramps should make you doubt pancreatitis
Serum lipase or amylase ≥ 3× the lab's upper limit of normal	**Lipase is preferred**—more sensitive, more specific, and remains elevated longer. Amylase is acceptable, but less reliable on its own—more prone to false positives and quicker to normalize.
Characteristic findings on CT, MRI, or (rarely) ultrasound	Cross-sectional imaging is mainly for diagnostic doubt or clinical decline; routine early CT is specifically discouraged

Our patient's pain is textbook, and her lipase is 15-fold normal, so she satisfies criteria 1 and 2 without a moment's hesitation. Because 2 criteria are already met, an immediate computed tomography (CT) would merely add cost and radiation without changing management. The guideline explicitly advises against "routine CT at admission" unless the story is murky or the patient fails to improve over the first 48-72 hours. Magnetic resonance imaging (MRI) is a reasonable alternative if imaging is truly needed—especially in patients with renal insufficiency or contrast allergy—but in a case like this, imaging adds no value.

Of course, telling that to the ED team doesn't always close the loop. These days, it can feel like anything from a stubbed toe to a sore throat warrants a CT abdomen "just to be sure." So even though the ACG is clear on this point, CTs still get ordered reflexively. That makes this a good teaching moment: if the patient has typical pancreatitis pain and a lipase (preferably) or amylase (still acceptable) ≥3× the ULN, then hold the scan and treat empirically. The pancreas doesn't need to be seen for AP to be believed.

> Routine CT is not required to diagnose AP in the setting of characteristic abdominal pain and either an elevated lipase or amylase ≥ 3x ULN

A few enzyme realities are worth remembering. First, the absence of a lipase bump does not rule out pancreatitis: up to one-fifth of alcohol-related or hypertriglyceridemic (HTG) AP cases present with a normal lipase. Remember that! It will come in handy. Conversely, amylase spikes can show up in salivary disease, renal failure, bowel ischemia, intestinal obstructions, macroamylasemia, or gynecological emergencies like ectopic pregnancy or tubo-ovarian abscesses, so lipase—not amylase—deserves top billing when you must pick 1 assay. Turns out the causes of high amylase spell out SALAMI, a food that doesn't cause pancreatitis but it's easy enough to remember (see **Figure 1.1**). Once the diagnosis is made, serial enzyme checks are unnecessary; trends do not predict severity, guide feeding, or influence discharge timing.[2]

> Remember that AP can present with a normal lipase

Figure 1.1. *Causes of High Amylase Spell out SALAMI.*

S alivary gland disease (parotitis, mumps, Sjögren's)

A cute pancreatitis

L ow GFR (renal failure)

A bdominal catastrophe (bowel ischemia, perf, SBO)

M acroamylasemia

I ntra-abdominal gyn emergency (ectopic, ovarian abscess)

Ultrasound's real purpose in the first hours is to detect gallstones, not to spell out pancreatic detail. Bowel gas often hides the gland; that limitation should not push the team toward a "better" CT if criteria are already satisfied. Imaging becomes useful only if the clinical course deviates from expectation: the patient deteriorates, fails to turn the corner by day 3, or presents with atypical pain and sub-diagnostic enzymes from the outset.

The next priority is early management—moderately aggressive hydration, preferably with lactated Ringer's (LR), along with pain control and vigilant monitoring of blood urea nitrogen, hematocrit, and any sign of systemic inflammatory response. More on management details in future vignettes.

Lactated Ringer's (LR) is preferred over normal saline for acute pancreatitis

But first, why LR? Here's why: Because it may reduce systemic inflammation more effectively than normal saline (NS). NS is slightly hyperchloremic and acidifying, which can worsen the metabolic acidosis often seen in pancreatitis, whereas LR is more balanced and less likely to exacerbate this physiologic stress.[3] Several trials have shown that LR can reduce SIRS scores and inflammatory markers in early AP.

In short, tell the ED: *She has acute pancreatitis; a scan tonight will not help her. Let's resuscitate, start guideline-directed care, and reserve cross-sectional imaging for uncertainty or complications.* With the diagnosis nailed down, the real detective work—why she developed pancreatitis and how to prevent complications—begins next.

So, let's continue the case with the next vignette.

Case 1.2: Six Hours Later...

You're back at the bedside of the 36-year-old woman with AP. It's now 6 hours after admission. Her nausea has improved, she's tolerating intravenous (IV) fluids (with LR, of course...), and her pain is better controlled. You confirmed the diagnosis based on her characteristic epigastric pain and markedly elevated lipase—no imaging was needed, despite the ED insisting it was necessary.

But now comes the next task: figuring out why she got pancreatitis in the first place.

She does not report a history of gallstone disease or prior similar episodes. She drinks alcohol socially, usually 1-2 drinks per week, but admits to "a few extra" the night before this episode—about 4 glasses of wine with dinner. No recent trauma, no new medications. Her body mass index (BMI) is 28. There's no family history of pancreatitis or early-onset diabetes.

Her abdominal ultrasound shows cholelithiasis but no gallbladder wall thickening, no pericholecystic fluid, and no bile duct dilation. The common bile duct measures 4 mm. Her alanine aminotransferase (ALT) is 28 U/L. Serum calcium is normal. Triglyceride levels are still pending.

Know your guidelines!

1. What does the ACG recommend as part of the initial etiologic workup for acute pancreatitis?

2. How do you interpret gallstones on ultrasound with a normal bile duct and normal liver tests?

3. When should you send for genetic testing or consider autoimmune pancreatitis?

4. What are the red flags for idiopathic pancreatitis that may not be so idiopathic after all?

Case 1.2: What do the guidelines say?

Source: ACG 2024 Acute Pancreatitis Guidelines[1]

The first order of business after you've diagnosed AP is to hunt down the trigger, because the ACG guideline remind us that most recurrences (and a fair bit of morbidity) are preventable once the culprit is exposed. The guideline lays out a straightforward, evidence-based template. Here are the highlights:

Start with the obvious. A careful history, basic chemistries, and a targeted ultrasound. Gallstones and alcohol together account for well over half of first attacks, so you always begin by asking about drinking patterns, scrutinizing old imaging when available, and—crucially—obtaining a high-quality transabdominal ultrasound. The guideline recommends everyone get that scan, and to repeat it if bowel gas or technique obscures the gallbladder or bile duct.[4]

> Everyone with acute pancreatitis needs an RUQ ultrasound (but not necessarily a CT)

Our patient's ultrasound does show stones, yet her duct is slender (4 mm) and her ALT is normal. That combination doesn't rule out biliary pancreatitis; tiny stones or sludge can pass transiently, inflame the pancreas, and leave only the gallbladder evidence behind. Because her bilirubin and duct are unremarkable, the ACG guidelines would not have us rush her to endoscopic retrograde cholangiopancreatography (ERCP), but they would still label this episode as "probable gallstone pancreatitis" and advise interval cholecystectomy once she stabilizes—otherwise her risk of a second attack is unacceptably high.[5]

> If gallstones are identified in AP, cholecystectomy is eventually warranted, even in the absence of an enlarged common bile duct

Screen for the metabolic imitators next. Draw a fasting triglyceride level and a serum calcium. HTG pancreatitis usually declares itself with triglyceride (TG) > 1,000 mg/dL, and hypercalcemia (think primary hyperparathyroidism or malignancy) is a rare but important reversible cause. If either value is abnormal, you've found your likely etiology; if they're normal, you move on.

When the first pass turns up nothing, escalate methodically—don't jump straight to labeling the case "idiopathic." The guideline's preferred ladder is repeat ultrasound or magnetic resonance cholangiopancreatography (MRCP), then (if still unrevealing) endoscopic ultrasound (EUS). EUS is remarkably sensitive for microlithiasis, small common duct stones, and early neoplasms, so in the modern era, "idiopathic" pancreatitis without an EUS or MRCP is really better described as "not yet looked for" pancreatitis.[6,7] Only after those imaging steps fail to explain the episode does the chart earn the "IAP" label.

Genetic and autoimmune workups are boutique tests, ordered for very specific scenarios—not routine day 1 labs. The guideline reserves genetic panels (*PRSS1, SPINK1, CFTR, CTRC*) for patients with recurrent unexplained attacks, a strong family history, or early-onset disease. We'll come back to those in a later vignettes but in this case it's premature to start ordering these tests. Likewise, autoimmune pancreatitis should only enter the differential if the imaging shows a sausage-shaped pancreas (more on that later, with fun pictures) or if there are systemic hints (obstructive jaundice with painless enlargement, salivary or lacrimal swelling, elevated immunoglobulin G4 [IgG4]). Ordering IgG4 blindly on every first-time AP admission merely adds noise. We'll come back to IgG4 later.

Only order genetic tests for recurrent unexplained AP, family history, and/or early-onset disease

So, what are the red flags that the pancreatitis called "idiopathic" might not be? Here are features that argue against using the term idiopathic: a second attack without a documented etiology; age >40 with unexplained weight loss (think occult pancreatic cancer); abnormal liver tests that spike then normalize (suggesting a passed stone); or persistent dilation of the pancreatic duct on follow-up imaging. Any one of those should send you back to MRCP or EUS before filing the case under "unknown."

In our patient, the working answer today is likely biliary: stones are present, nothing else has surfaced, and we've ordered the TG level to be sure. If the TGs return <150 mg/dL and she remains stone-positive but duct-normal, the plan is straightforward—laparoscopic cholecystectomy once she's recovered, and no ERCP unless jaundice or cholangitis appears. Should the ultrasound have been equivocal or stone-free, MRCP (or better, EUS) would be next. Only after negative advanced imaging, normal TG and calcium, no suspicious medications, and no excessive alcohol would we let her carry the "idiopathic" tag—and even then we'd keep one eyebrow raised for a silent tumor or occult gallstone disease on future imaging.

Bottom line: The 2024 ACG pathway is deliberately simple—ultrasound to look for stones, labs for alcohol-independent metabolic triggers, repeat or advanced imaging if nothing clicks, and reserve the esoteric tests for special circumstances. Follow that algorithm and very few "mystery" pancreatitis cases stay mysterious for long.

Case 1.3: The Next 48 Hours

It's now day 2 of hospitalization for your 36-year-old patient with AP, likely biliary in origin. She was started on IV LR at 150 mL/hour on admission, received an initial 1L bolus in the ED, and was transitioned to patient-controlled analgesia (PCA) with morphine overnight. Her vitals have remained stable, but she's still having moderate abdominal pain and some lingering nausea. Her intake has been minimal. The team kept her nil per os (NPO) "until pain improved," but she's now asking when she can try some water or maybe even something light. Her abdomen remains tender in the epigastrium but without guarding or rebound. She has not vomited overnight.

Labs this morning show: blood urea nitrogen (BUN): 22 mg/dL (was 17 on admission); hematocrit (HCT): 43% (was 39%); WBC: 14.2; Creatinine (Cr): 1.1 (baseline 0.8); no signs of systemic inflammatory response syndrome (SIRS) or organ dysfunction.

The hospitalist asks: Should we keep pushing fluids at this rate? Is this patient developing severe pancreatitis? And is it okay to let her eat?

Know your guidelines!

1. How do you manage IV fluids in the first 48 hours of AP—and when do you hold back?
2. What signs should alert you that the patient is getting worse?
3. Is there any role for scoring systems like Ranson, BISAP, or APACHE in guiding severity or care?
4. When should oral intake be resumed, and do we still need to "wait for pain to resolve" or lipase to normalize?
5. Do you give prophylactic antibiotics in patients who remain febrile or have leukocytosis?

Case 1.3: What do the guidelines say?
Source: ACG 2024 Acute Pancreatitis Guidelines[1]

Early management of AP is where missteps magnify into morbidity, so let's walk through what the 2024 ACG guideline expects us to do—and also what it asks us not to do—over the first 48 hours. Following these critical guidelines can save lives.

Fluids: "Moderately Aggressive," Not a Fire Hose

> Watch the delta BUN and delta HCT carefully during initial management of AP. If both are positive, the patient is not adequately hydrated

She has already received a 1 liter bolus plus LR at 150 mL/h. Yet her BUN has crept from 17 → 22 mg/dL and her hematocrit from 39 → 43%. That's not good. Always keep an eye out on the delta BUN and delta HCT; they can give you a quick assessment of whether you're keeping up with third spacing. Rising hemoconcentration despite fluids is the guideline's red flag that perfusion is still inadequate and the pancreas may be headed toward necrosis if underperfusion continues.

That said, before you reflexively double the drip and blast away with LR, pause long enough to look for volume-overload risk—heart failure, renal compromise, baseline oxygen requirement—but in an otherwise healthy 36-year-old you can safely step up to 2-3 mL/kg/h for the next 4-6 hours, recheck BUN/HCT, and back down as soon as those numbers stabilize or fall. The key is to constantly monitor for adequacy of resuscitation; don't just set an LR rate and leave for the night. Sign out this sort of thing with a clear action plan. Watch carefully, and then apply the rules shown in **Table 1.2**, and tweak the fluids accordingly.

Remember that LR remains the fluid of choice: as we covered earlier, this solution is less acidifying than NS, better preserves microcirculatory flow, and in randomized, controlled trials (RCTs) lowered early SIRS scores compared with saline.

That leads to the next point: What's a SIRS score, and why do we care? SIRS stands for Systemic Inflammatory Response Syndrome, and

Table 1.2. *Bedside markers that tell you your fluids are working—or failing.*

Trend in First 24h	Interpretation	Recommended Tweak
BUN falling or steady	Good: Renal perfusion adequate	Continue current fluid rate
BUN rising ≥ 5 mg/dL	Bad: Patient is under-resuscitated	Bolus 10 mL/Kg, increase rate, and recheck in 4-6 hours
Hematocrit drifting towards 35%-44%	Good: Hemodilution is on track	Maintain current fluid strategy
Hematocrit climbing >44%	Bad: Hemoconcentration	Same as for rising BUN: bolus and reassess volume status
Peripheral edema, crackles, high O2 need	Bad: Volume overload	Slow or pause infusion; consider diuresis if needed

it's a simple, bedside-friendly way to gauge whether inflammation is spilling beyond the pancreas into systemic territory. You get 1 point for each of the following:

- Temperature >100.9°F or <96.8°F
- Heart rate >90 bpm
- Respiratory rate >20 breaths/min* or $PaCO_2$ <32 mmHg
- WBC >12,000 or <4,000, or >10% bands

A SIRS score of ≥2 suggests early systemic inflammation, and persistent SIRS (lasting beyond 48 hours) is a strong predictor of more severe disease. That's why the ACG guideline recommends monitoring these values closely during the initial 24-48 hours. While it's not a perfect tool, SIRS gives us real-time clues that the inflammatory process might be escalating, and that's exactly where smart fluid management—and early feeding—can make a difference.

* Do you ever notice that even stable patients seem to have a respiratory rate of 20 routinely marked in the chart? Author B.S. has a rule: If the respiratory rate is a multiple of 5, it might not be real. Check for yourself! Remember that 20 is fast, which is why it's considered a marker of severity in the SIRS scoring system.

Severity: Read the Patient, Not Just the Score

Her vitals are stable, she has no organ failure, and she hasn't met SIRS criteria—so for now, she sits squarely in the "mild" acute pancreatitis bucket. Some clinicians might calculate a BISAP score here—and that's fine, as long as you know what it is and what it isn't. BISAP stands for **B**edside **I**ndex for **S**everity in **A**cute **P**ancreatitis, and it gives 1 point each for the following 5 findings within 24 hours of presentation:

- **B**UN >25 mg/dL
- **I**mpaired mental status (Glasgow Coma Scale <15)
- **S**IRS (≥2 criteria)
- **A**ge >60
- **P**leural effusion on imaging

Our patient would score 1 for SIRS (white count >12,000), but that's not especially worrisome in isolation. The real utility of BISAP is in identifying patients at risk for complications or death—a score ≥3 is associated with worse outcomes.[8] But the ACG is clear: 1-time scores should never override clinical judgment.[9] The real danger signal is persistent organ failure lasting more than 48 hours—that's when a patient graduates to severe acute pancreatitis and probably needs Intensive Care Unit (ICU)-level care. Until then, trending the basics—BUN, hematocrit, urine output, SIRS criteria—is a more valuable compass than any 5-point index.

A BISAP score >3 predicts mortality in AP

"Can I Eat Yet?" — Yes, Sooner Than You Might Think

The old "NPO until pain-free" dogma is gone. Many of us learned in med school to "let the pancreas rest," as if it's just too tired to be pushed, and tweaking it with a meal might lead to catastrophe. Turns out that was wrong. Multiple trials show that early oral feeding—within 24 to 48 hours—shortens length of stay, improves outcomes, and does not increase complications, even in patients with ongoing pain.[10] Because she is hemodynamically stable and no longer vomiting, she's

Early oral feeding in AP shortens length of stay, improves clinical outcomes, and does not increase risk of complications a perfect candidate to try eating. Start with a low-fat solid meal or whatever bland entrée the kitchen can muster—there's no need to tiptoe through clear liquids. If she belches twice and feels queasy, simply pause and retry in a few hours—no harm done.

If she remains unable to tolerate oral intake by 72 hours, that's when you pivot to enteral nutrition—preferably via nasogastric (NG) tube. The guideline is clear that NG and nasojejunal (NJ) routes are equally effective and safe, and NG is far easier to place.[11] There's no need to reflexively bypass the stomach unless the patient has severe gastroparesis, refractory vomiting, or very high aspiration risk. NJ tubes are reserved for those rare cases (despite a strong yet incorrect drive by some to always place an NJ, which is not supported by data). Parenteral nutrition should remain a last resort, reserved only for patients who absolutely cannot tolerate enteral feeding despite multiple attempts.

> If patient cannot tolerate POs after 72 hours, then start enteral. NG is easier to place than NJ and there's no difference in outcomes

In short: feed early, feed enterally whenever possible, and don't get fancy with the route unless you have to. Oral is always preferred. The pancreas is more resilient than we once thought—it can handle a meal. While on the topic of oral feeds, we wanted to introduce the Karsan Tray Sign, which we utilize on hospital rounds to help determine when it's time for discharge. We check the food tray on rounds, and if the plate is clean (i.e., the patient has eaten everything in sight), then you have a positive Karsan Tray Sign, indicating that the patient is ready for discharge home. Nearly a 100% positive predictive value!

Antibiotics: Still a Firm *No* in Uncomplicated Early AP

Her leukocytosis is almost certainly inflammatory, not infectious—which is common in early pancreatitis and not a reason to jump immediately to antibiotics. The ACG guideline is unequivocal here: prophylactic antibiotics do not prevent infection of necrotic tissue, do not reduce mortality, and should not be used routinely. This is one of the more persistent myths in pancreatitis management—that a rising WBC or fever in the first few days must mean infection and

Routine antibiotics are not recommended in AP. But use if there are gas bubbles in a necrotic collection or infection on an aspirate

should be met with a broad-spectrum antibiotic "just in case." But in AP, systemic inflammation alone can drive fever, leukocytosis, and even SIRS without a single microbe involved. That's why the guidelines recommend holding off on antibiotics unless there's clear evidence of infection.[12,13] What counts as clear evidence? Think positive cultures, gas bubbles in necrotic collections on imaging, or a positive aspirate from CT- or EUS-guided fine needle aspiration (FNA). Without one of those, you're treating inflammation with unnecessary antibiotics—which only breeds resistance, invites *Clostridioides difficile*, and clouds the picture.

If antibiotics are warranted, use either a carbapenem or fluoroquinolone + metronidazole

When true infected necrosis is confirmed, then and only then is it time to start appropriate therapy. The guidelines recommend coverage with a carbapenem, or a fluoroquinolone plus metronidazole, because these agents have reliable penetration into necrotic pancreatic tissue. We'll come back to this situation in a forthcoming vignette.

The takeaway for this case is simple but important: elevated WBC does not equal infection in pancreatitis. You're treating the pancreas, not the white count. Hold the antibiotics until you have something real to treat.

Bringing It Together

1. **Fluids.** Increase LR to ~250 mL/h (≈ 3 mL/kg/h) for 6 hours, recheck BUN/HCT; back off once the numbers fall or if pulmonary exam worsens.
2. **Pain**. Keep PCA morphine; titrate to comfort, no evidence that opioids worsen course.
3. **Feed early and often**. Offer a low-fat solid breakfast today. If tolerated, advance diet. Don't get all worried that eating a meal will destroy the pancreas. It won't.
4. **Monitor**. Vitals every 4h, I/O, BUN, HCT every 6-8h for the first 24h, then daily if stable.

5. **No empiric antibiotics, no CT scan**. Unless clinical deterioration demands it.

If her labs stabilize and she tolerates food, she'll meet "mild AP" criteria and could be ready for discharge by day 3 with a plan for interval laparoscopic cholecystectomy. Should organ failure blossom or her BUN continues to climb despite fluids, you'll escalate to ICU monitoring and reevaluate for early complications—but you are now following the ACG playbook to the letter, and that's exactly where she needs you to be.

Case 1.4: Something's Brewing

A 58-year-old man with obesity and well-controlled type 2 diabetes presents with 3 days of severe epigastric pain radiating to the back, nausea, and subjective fevers. He drinks alcohol occasionally but denies recent binges. Vitals on admission: temperature 100.8°F, heart rate (HR) 108, blood pressure (BP) 116/72, respiratory rate (RR) 20, O_2 sat 96% on room air. He is tender in the epigastrium without rebound. Lipase is 980 U/L, BUN is 27, Cr 1.3 (baseline 1.0), and WBC 15.6. Transaminases are normal. Triglycerides are mildly elevated at 260 mg/dL.

He is admitted with a diagnosis of AP and started on IV LR, bowel rest, and pain control. But by hospital day 3, he still has persistent fevers, worsening abdominal pain, and now requires supplemental oxygen. His BUN is climbing despite fluids.

You order a CT scan with contrast, which reveals pancreatic and peripancreatic fluid collections with areas of non-enhancement involving over 30% of the gland. There's no obvious gas in the collection.

Surgery is consulted and suggests early percutaneous drainage "to be proactive." The hospitalist asks whether antibiotics are now indicated "just in case." The team looks to you.

Know your guidelines!

1. When should necrosis be suspected in acute pancreatitis?
2. How do you distinguish acute necrotic collection from a pseudocyst or simple fluid?
3. What defines infected necrosis, and how do you diagnose it?
4. Should this patient get antibiotics?
5. When is the right time to drain a necrotic collection?

Case 1.4: What do the guidelines say?

Source: ACG 2024 Acute Pancreatitis Guidelines[1]

Whereas the earlier patient fell in the mild end of the spectrum, this patient reminds us why pancreatitis can still keep us up at night. Three days in, his clinical picture (persistent fever, worsening pain, creeping BUN/Cr, new O_2 need) says "not mild." A contrast CT confirms it: patchy, non-enhancing parenchyma with shaggy peripancreatic fluid—acute necrotic collection (ANC) involving > 30% of the gland. **Figure 1.2** shows the classic appearance.

Figure 1.2. *Acute Necrotic Collection in AP. Axial CT showing hypoenhancement of the pancreas (white solid arrows) and free fluid in the abdomen (white dashed arrow), consistent with acute necrotizing pancreatitis.*[14]

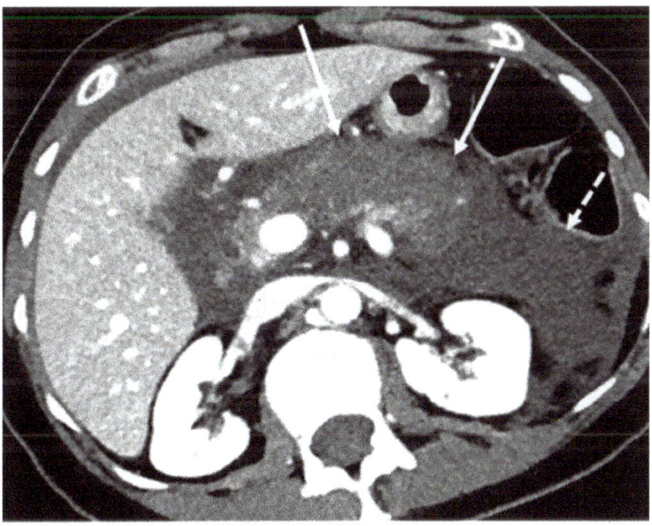

Necrosis ≠ Automatic Intervention

Early pancreatic necrosis is almost always sterile

Keep in mind that early necrosis is almost always sterile and usually behaves if you control the systemic threats. Less than one-third of ANC ever requires drainage—what pushes the rest over the cliff is hypoperfusion, unbridled SIRS, or secondary infection. That's why the ACG guideline's prime directive is supportive stewardship first, procedures later.

Recognizing the 4 Collection Types

Before we decide how to manage a pancreatic or peripancreatic fluid collection, we need to know exactly what we're looking at—and that starts with speaking the right language.

The Revised Atlanta Classification, which the ACG guideline adopts, was created to bring clarity and standardization to the often-confusing world of pancreatitis-related collections.[15] Rather than lumping everything under vague terms like "phlegmon" or "abscess," it defines 4 specific types of collections, based on their timing, content, and whether or not they have a defined wall. Understanding this framework is crucial because each type carries different clinical implications, particularly regarding the need for drainage or surgery. The classifications are broken down in **Table 1.3**.

Table 1.3. *Four types of pancreatic fluid collections.*

Collection type	Contents	Wall present	Typical timing
Acute peripancreatic fluid collection (APFC)	Pure fluid	No	<4 wk
Acute necrotic collection (ANC)	Fluid ± solid debris	No	<4 wk
Pseudocyst	Pure fluid	Yes	≥ 4 wk
Walled-off necrosis (WON)	Fluid + necrotic debris	Yes	≥ 4 wk

APFC is what you see in uncomplicated interstitial pancreatitis. It's bland, sterile fluid that almost always resolves on its own.

ANC means dead tissue is now in the mix. It may liquefy over time, but in the first few weeks, it's mostly a soup of fluid and sloughed-off parenchyma. Lovely.

Pseudocysts form when pure fluid persists long enough (≥ 4 weeks) to develop a defined capsule. These are common in patients with prior mild or moderate pancreatitis. Remember that it's called a "pseudo" cyst to distinguish it from a real cyst. That's because a real cyst has an epithelialized capsule, whereas a pseudocyst does not. Instead, the capsule is just super compressed pancreatic parenchyma from the squeeze of the accumulated fluid, but it's not a true cyst. Moreover, that lack of epithelium is also why there's no risk of malignancy for a pseudocyst.

WON is the mature form of ANC—same nasty ingredients (fluid and solid debris), but now surrounded by a fibrous wall, making it safer to access if drainage becomes necessary.

Understanding these distinctions matters. You don't drain collections just because they exist—you drain them when they're infected or symptomatic, and when they're organized enough to allow it. That means timing is everything. Trying to intervene too early—before a wall forms—is often more dangerous than doing nothing at all.

> Not every fluid collection in the pancreas needs to be drained. Be careful not to drain prematurely or things can go from bad to worse

Is It Infected?

One of the most critical decisions you'll face with necrotizing pancreatitis is determining whether the necrosis has become infected. It's tempting to reach for antibiotics early—especially when the patient has leukocytosis and persistent fevers—but the ACG guideline is unambiguous: don't treat a number. Not every fever in pancreatitis is infectious, and not every necrosis needs antibiotics. So, what actually counts as infection? The guideline offers 3 specific scenarios that justify treatment:

1. Gas bubbles visible within the collection on CT—this is the most specific sign.
2. Positive culture from FNA, if obtained.
3. Clinical signs of sepsis with no other source—e.g., hypotension, rigors, or worsening organ dysfunction that can't be explained otherwise.

In our case, none of those are present. He has leukocytosis, but that's expected in this phase. No gas is seen on imaging. He's uncomfortable, yes, but stable. This is not the time to pull the antibiotic trigger. Starting broad-spectrum antibiotics now doesn't reduce the risk of infection later, and it may do more harm than good. You increase the chance of drug resistance, *C. difficile*, and you make any future culture results uninterpretable.

Instead, closely monitor. If he deteriorates—develops new fevers, signs of shock, or rising procalcitonin—you reassess. But until then, the antibiotics stay on the shelf.

Should We Drain Now?

Short answer? *No.*

Even though the CT shows necrosis involving more than 30% of the gland, that's not a reason to intervene in isolation. The ACG guideline, backed by multiple RCTs, strongly discourages early drainage or debridement in the absence of confirmed or strongly suspected infection, or life-threatening complications (such as abdominal compartment syndrome or refractory organ failure).

Why wait? Because early necrotic collections—like the ANC in our patient—are disorganized and gelatinous. There's no clean wall, no drainage tract, and no safe plane for debridement. Trying to poke it now creates more problems: bleeding, fistulae, and incomplete clearance that leads to chronic sepsis.

Intervention should be delayed at least 4 weeks, if possible, to allow the collection to mature into WON. At that point, the liquefied contents can be more easily drained, and the fibrous wall makes percutaneous or endoscopic approaches safer and more effective.

> Attempting to drain a fluid collection without a wall can lead to bleeding, fistula, and incomplete clearance. Try to wait 4 weeks before draining if possible

What if the patient crashes? That's different. If infection is confirmed and the patient is septic, then the approach is step-up drainage, starting with percutaneous or endoscopic drainage first, not surgery. Open necrosectomy is reserved for the rare case where everything else fails.

So, despite the surgical consult's eagerness to "get ahead of it," the right move is supportive care and watchful waiting—not proactive poking.

What Defines Severity Now?

This is a good time to pause and reemphasize that severe AP is not defined by imaging findings. The amount of necrosis is important, yes—but what really matters is organ failure. According to the revised Atlanta classification,[15] adopted by the ACG guideline:

- **Mild AP** = no organ failure, no complications;
- **Moderately severe AP** = transient organ failure (< 48h) or local/systemic complications without persistent organ failure;
- **Severe AP** = persistent organ failure (> 48h) affecting 1 or more organs.

So even though this patient has necrosis, if his kidney function improves with fluids and his oxygen needs stabilize, he remains in the moderately severe camp. If he worsens and needs pressors, dialysis, or ventilatory support beyond 48 hours, then we upgrade to severe AP, and everything changes.

Your Move: Supportive Care, Not Intervention

So, what should you do now? In short, **support, observe, and don't rush in.**

- Hold antibiotics unless infection is confirmed—fever and leukocytosis (which are components of SIRS) alone aren't enough.
- Continue careful fluid management, adjusting based on BUN, hematocrit, and clinical status (**Table 1.2**).
- Initiate enteral nutrition if oral intake remains inadequate by day 4—NG is fine; no need to go NJ unless there is a clear reason.
- Monitor for evolving organ failure—persistent organ dysfunction > 48 hours reclassifies this as severe AP.
- Plan repeat imaging only if he clinically worsens or fails to improve by 7–10 days; otherwise, reassess around week 4 to

evaluate for wall formation.

- Engage your multidisciplinary team early, but be clear: no drainage, no debridement—not yet.

Let the collection mature, keep the patient stable, and reserve interventions for when they're truly needed—and safer to perform. This is the moment where doing less actually is doing more.

Bottom line: This case is the perfect reminder that restraint is a therapeutic choice. Just because necrosis is present doesn't mean that something has to be done—yet. The guideline urges us to manage physiologic instability first, give the body time to do its work, and only intervene when the benefit is clear.

Support now. Drain later. Poke last.

Case 1.5: A Hot Mess in Week 3

It's now hospital day 18 for the 58-year-old man you admitted with severe AP and pancreatic necrosis. You initially managed him conservatively per guidelines—no early drainage, no antibiotics, and close ICU monitoring. He stabilized on fluids, required short-term oxygen, and tolerated a trickle of NG feeds. But this week, something changed.

He's had persistent low-grade fevers the past 3 days, which were initially attributed to central line colonization—but now he's spiking to 102.9°F. His heart rate is in the 110s, his WBC has climbed to 18.2, and he's looking more uncomfortable. BUN is stable, but he's more tachypneic and requires supplemental oxygen again.

A repeat contrast-enhanced CT scan shows an evolving walled-off necrotic collection in the left anterior pararenal space. It now measures 12 cm, and there's a visible gas bubble inside. The radiology report adds, "consistent with infected necrosis."

Know your guidelines!

1. How is infected necrosis defined on imaging or clinically?
2. Do we need an FNA before starting antibiotics?
3. When—and by what route—should drainage be performed?
4. What is the proper step-up approach, and how do we decide between percutaneous, endoscopic, or surgical options?
5. Is it ever appropriate to treat with antibiotics alone?

Case 1.5: What do the guidelines say?

Source: ACG 2024 Acute Pancreatitis Guidelines[1]

By week 3, a necrotic pancreas can smolder quietly—or tip into frank sepsis.* The ACG guidelines draws a line between **sterile** and **infected** necrosis, because management flips the instant infection is judged "overwhelmingly likely." Our patient just crossed that line.

So, how do we know if this is this truly infected necrosis? As mentioned in the earlier vignettes (but worth repeating here), the ACG guidelines accept any 1 of 3 proofs:

1. **Gas bubbles** inside the walled-off necrosis on CT or MRI (**Figure 1.3** shows the classic "streak of air" sign).
2. **Positive culture** from CT-guided FNA.
3. **Clinical sepsis and necrosis** on imaging when no other source explains the deterioration.

Figure 1.3. *Gas bubbles in a necrotic pancreas – not good. Abdominal CT showing the "streak of air sign" (arrow) in emphysematous pancreatitis due to significant pancreatic and peripancreatic gas-containing fluid collection.*[16]

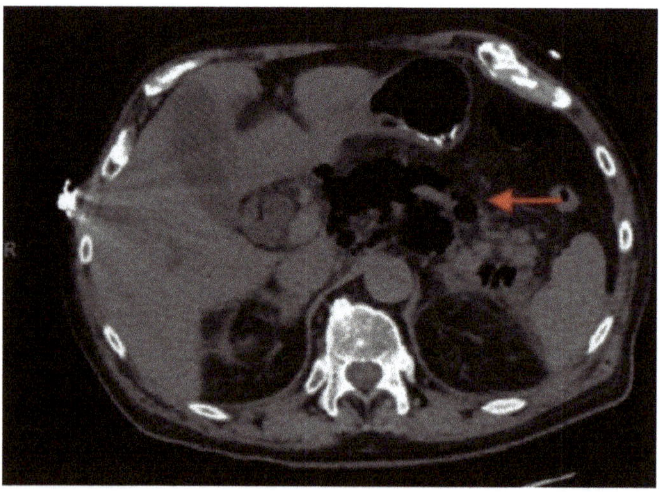

This patient has new SIRS physiology and visible intralesional gas, so

* Who is this guy "Frank" who always gets sepsis?

he has met criteria without needing an FNA. When imaging already shows gas, the authors state bluntly: skip the needle, start the drugs.

Next Step: Start Antibiotics Now—What & Why

Empiric therapy must reach the poorly perfused necrotic core. Carbapenems (imipenem, meropenem) have the best penetration; a fluoroquinolone plus metronidazole is an acceptable alternative if *Pseudomonas* coverage is not required. Cultures from blood, prior drains, or (if you still choose) FNA can later tailor the regimen, but delay is the enemy.[17] The guideline emphasizes: that antibiotics are therapeutic, not prophylactic; they belong only when infection is proven or virtually certain, as it is today for this patient.

Carbapenems have the best penetration into necrotic pancreas

Should you drain now or wait? Early, open necrosectomy is history—mortality drops when we delay any instrumentation until a fibrous wall matures, usually ≈4 weeks after onset. That interval lets liquefaction occur and separates dead from viable tissue, turning a shredding debridement into a tidy scoop-and-suction. So it's premature to start manipulating the pancreas if you can otherwise avoid it. As the surgeons know best, don't mess with the pancreas if you don't need to; it can cause more harm than good.

While we wait to see what happens next, 1 of 2 pathways may emerge, as shown in **Table 1.4**.

Table 1.4. *What to do after starting antibiotics for infected pancreatic necrosis.*

Patient trajectory	Next move
Hemodynamically stable after antibiotics; organ function improving	Continue antibiotics alone, reassess twice weekly; up to ~50 % clear infection without drainage
Persistent sepsis, organ failure, enlarging or symptomatic collection	Begin step-up drainage immediately

The modern "step-up" approach for this situation is deliberately slow and measured—each maneuver buys time for the next, more

If sepsis persists despite antibiotics, start with percutaneous catheter drainage

aggressive rung only if the patient refuses to improve. If sepsis persists, then percutaneous catheter drainage (PCD) should be placed under CT or ultrasound guidance. A 12- to 14-Fr pigtail is usually sufficient; it can be upsized or multiplied later. Roughly half of patients declared "infected" will defervesce, watch their white count fall, and turn the clinical corner with nothing more than PCD plus targeted antibiotics. Daily saline flushes keep the catheter patent, and serial CT every week or two confirms that the cavity is shrinking rather than compartmentalizing.

If, after 48-72 hours, fever, pain, or organ failure refuse to relent, the guideline's next rung is endoscopic transluminal therapy. Under EUS guidance, a lumen-apposing metal stent (LAMS) is fired across the gastric or duodenal wall, creating a 10-15 mm conduit into the walled-off necrosis. Thick debris is lavaged through the stent; the endoscopist may return every few days with a standard or pediatric scope to retrieve non-liquefied chunks—a minimally invasive necrosectomy performed entirely through the stomach, which has been shown to improve outcomes compared with surgical necrosectomy.[18]

If PCD fails, then move next to LAMS, not straight to necrosectomy

Surgical debridement. Only when percutaneous tubes and repeated endoscopic sessions fail—or when anatomy simply blocks a safe trans-gastric route—do we escalate to surgical debridement. Even then, the knife is kept small: video-assisted retroperitoneal debridement or laparoscopic transperitoneal approaches are preferred, reserving open necrosectomy for the rare patient whose disease or prior operations preclude minimal access. The key principle is sequential escalation: **tube first, scope second, scalpel last**—always letting each step declare success or failure before climbing higher.

A succinct way to remember timing:

Antibiotics first → stick a percutaneous drain if still sick → scope if drain under-performs → knife only after scopes fail.

If the patient stabilizes while on antibiotics—that is, they defervesce, the WBC drops, and organ support is not needed—you should continue IV antibiotics 2-3 weeks, then switch to an oral agent with good bioavailability (e.g., levofloxacin + metronidazole) to complete a 4- to 6-week course. Serial CT or MRI every 2–3 weeks tracks cavity size; residual sterile "cold WON" rarely needs intervention.

Bringing It Together

1. Start meropenem immediately; obtain blood cultures but don't wait on growth.
2. Alert interventional radiology; place a 12- to 14-Fr percutaneous drain into the gas-containing collection today.
3. Begin daily drain irrigation and watch vitals, urine output, lactate.
4. If he is still febrile or pressor-dependent at 72 h, move to endoscopic LAMS-guided necrosectomy.
5. Keep the surgeons in the loop—but they stay on the bench unless minimally invasive steps fail.

With that sequence, the guideline shows mortality under 10%, a stunning improvement over the bad old days of early open necrosectomy. Patience, good drains, and the right antibiotics save more pancreases—and patients—than the scalpel.

Case 1.6: Rock and Roll

A 62-year-old woman with a history of hypertension and hyperlipidemia presents with sudden onset epigastric pain radiating to her back, associated with nausea and vomiting. She ate a double cheeseburger last night at a Pearl Jam concert and awoke with intense, persistent upper abdominal pain early this morning. In the ED, she is afebrile but mildly tachycardic. On exam, she is tender in the epigastrium and right upper quadrant (RUQ), without guarding or rebound.

Initial labs reveal: WBC: 13.8; Lipase: 1150 U/L; ALT: 268 U/L; aspartate aminotransferase (AST): 198 U/L; alkaline phosphatase (ALP): 188 U/L; Total bilirubin: 3.1 mg/dL; Direct bilirubin: 2.4 mg/dL.

An RUQ ultrasound reveals cholelithiasis with a mildly dilated common bile duct (CBD) measuring 8 mm. No gallbladder wall thickening or pericholecystic fluid is seen. The pancreas is partially obscured.

The ED team calls you to admit her for gallstone pancreatitis. They ask if you want to get an MRCP... or should she go straight to ERCP?

Know your guidelines!

1. What are the indications for ERCP in acute biliary pancreatitis?
2. How do you distinguish choledocholithiasis from cholangitis, and why does it matter?
3. When is MRCP or EUS appropriate, and how should these tests be sequenced?
4. Is ERCP ever done "just in case" in biliary pancreatitis?

Case 1.6: What do the guidelines say?

Source: ACG 2024 Acute Pancreatitis Guidelines[1]

Gallstone pancreatitis is a double-edged sword: you must tame the inflamed pancreas *and* decide whether a rogue common duct stone is still obstructing the ampulla. The ACG guidelines wants to ensure we do not swing that ductal sword prematurely. (Okay, this analogy isn't perfect...) Let's walk through its logic step by step.

First Question: Is this cholangitis?

The only truly "stat" indication for ERCP in acute biliary pancreatitis is suspected or confirmed cholangitis. But cholangitis is more than just a bump in bilirubin—it's a systemic infection of the biliary tree, and the stakes are high. The classic clinical clue is Charcot's triad: fever, right upper quadrant pain, and jaundice. If you're truly unlucky, you get the full house—Reynolds' pentad—which adds hypotension and altered mental status to the mix and signals impending septic shock. That's not good. These aren't just board buzzwords; they guide real-world decisions, especially when imaging lags or labs are equivocal.

Charcot's triad:

* Fever
* RUQ pain
* Jaundice

Add hypotension and AMS and you get Reynold's pentad

Our patient, however, is afebrile, hemodynamically stable, alert, and her leukocytosis is modest at 13.8. She has RUQ tenderness and a bilirubin of 3.1, but that doesn't make cholangitis. Without systemic toxicity or signs of sepsis, the ACG guideline makes a strong recommendation: hold the ERCP until you know there's actually a stone to retrieve.

Second Question: How likely is a stone still in the duct?

To help determine the need for ERCP, shown in **Figure 1.4**, we can utilize the high/intermediate/low probability framework from the ASGE guideline.[19] Stones flagged on imaging, or ascending colangitis, or a bilirubin over 4 mg/dL plus a dilated duct, place the patient in the high-probability category and justify direct ERCP. But this patient has an 8-mm CBD and bilirubin 3.1 mg/dL—squarely intermediate risk. Data tell us that two-thirds of such patients have already dropped their stone into the duodenum by the time the scope gets to the papilla; proceeding straight to ERCP would expose her to risk with no payoff most of the time.[20] The guideline therefore strongly recommends non-invasive confirmation first.

Figure 1.4. *Management pathway for suspected CBD stone in biliary pancreatitis.*[19]

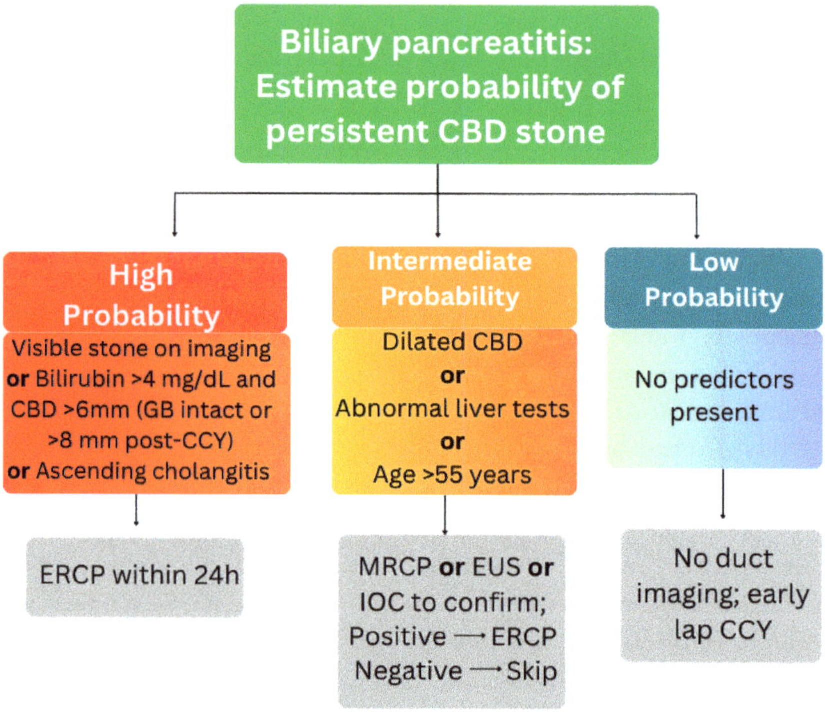

Third Question: MRCP or EUS as the gatekeeper?

Either modality is north of 95% sensitive for stones 5 mm or larger. If you can do a same-session EUS-then-ERCP under 1 anesthetic, that is efficient. In many U.S. hospitals, however, EUS capacity is limited, or scheduling delays defeat the purpose; in those settings an MRCP obtained from radiology within a few hours becomes the practical choice. What matters is to keep up the pace and follow the guidance in **Figure 1.4**. If MRCP gets you there faster, then go for it. If the MRCP shows choledocholithiasis, as in **Figure 1.5**, then you would need to clear the duct with ERCP. Otherwise, if the MRCP or intraoperative cholangiogram (IOC) is negative, there is no need to be an ERCP hero.

Figure 1.5. *MRCP showing 2 distal CBD stones (arrow).*

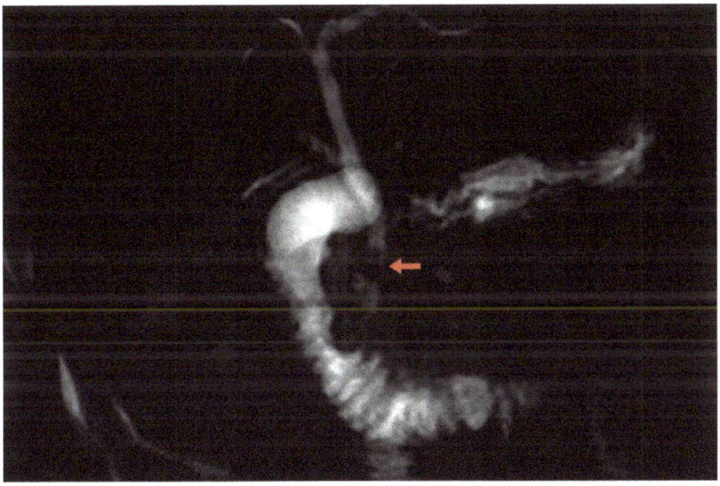

Fourth Question: When does cholecystectomy happen?

For mild gallstone pancreatitis, the answer is "this admission." Same-stay laparoscopic cholecystectomy slashes the risk of recurrent pancreatitis or cholangitis by more than half and saves the healthcare system readmission dollars.[21] Clearing the duct with an ERCP does not remove the gallbladder from the OR schedule; it only settles today's crisis.

> Gallstone pancreatitis should lead to same-admission cholecystectomy if possible

Fifth Question: What about PEP prophylaxis if she does reach ERCP?

PEP stands for post-ERCP pancreatitis—the most common and feared complication of the procedure, occurring in roughly 5% of average-risk patients and up to 20% of high-risk cases. Two preventive measures have the strongest evidence base and are baked into the guideline:

Always check for NSAID allergy before packing the rectum with indomethacin!

- **Rectal indomethacin 100 mg** given immediately before—or at the latest within 30 minutes after—scope withdrawal. Multiple RCTs and meta-analyses show a single suppository slices PEP risk roughly in half. ***Critical caveat:*** always confirm there's no history of aspirin or non-steroidal anti-inflammatory drug (NSAID) allergy or severe NSAID-related asthma before the patient drifts off under sedation; once the propofol is flowing, it's too late to get a reliable history, and a well-intended dose can end in bronchospasm or anaphylaxis.
- **Vigorous periprocedural hydration with LR** (e.g., 3 mL/kg/h during the case plus a 20 mL/kg bolus afterward). Small but well-designed trials demonstrate lower enzyme peaks and fewer admissions when LR accompanies indomethacin and has been recommended.[22]

A prophylactic pancreatic duct stent is now reserved for situations that intrinsically jack up risk—prolonged or traumatic cannulation, need for precut access, pancreatic sphincter balloon work, ampullectomy, or other complex maneuvers. When indomethacin and generous LR are delivered reliably, routine "just in case" stenting of otherwise low-risk ducts is no longer recommended.

Bringing It Together

1. No emergency ERCP tonight—she lacks cholangitis.
2. Order MRCP (or EUS if available on short notice) to confirm or refute a retained CBD stone. (Isn't MRCP the best, by the way? Love that test.)
3. Positive study? ERCP within 24 hours, with indomethacin and LR hydration.
4. Negative study? Skip ERCP, manage the pancreatitis medically, and schedule laparoscopic cholecystectomy before discharge.
5. Once her pain resolves and labs trend down, send her home stone-free and gallbladder-free, minimizing her chance of an encore hospital performance. Rather, she'll be able to go to more

live Pearl Jam encore performances, which sounds a lot better!

Pearl Jam is one of the best rock bands of all time and puts on a great live performance!

By forcing us to prove ductal obstruction rather than assume it, the ACG guideline prevents 2 out of 3 patients like her from undergoing an unnecessary ERCP—yet still protects the one who truly needs urgent biliary decompression. It is a perfect example of evidence shaping precision care: intervene only when benefit is proven, not presumed.

Case 1.7: Here We Go Again

A 40-year-old man presents with his third episode of AP in the last 18 months. Each episode has followed the same script: sudden onset epigastric pain radiating to the back, associated with nausea and vomiting. His lipase today is 1,450 U/L, and he meets full diagnostic criteria for acute pancreatitis.

He denies alcohol use and has no history of gallstones. His BMI is 24. He is not on any new medications and has no known family history of pancreatic disease. He does not smoke or use recreational drugs.

Labs today show: WBC: 12.6; ALT: 28 U/L; AST: 31 U/L; ALP: 82 U/L; Total bilirubin: 0.9 mg/dL; Triglycerides: 146 mg/dL; Calcium: 9.4 mg/dL.

An ultrasound during his first episode showed no gallstones and a normal common bile duct. He had a contrast-enhanced CT during his second episode, which showed mild interstitial pancreatitis and no collections or masses. No MRCP or EUS has been done to date. The admitting hospitalist writes "idiopathic pancreatitis" as the admitting diagnosis and calls you for help.

Know your guidelines!

1. What constitutes a complete workup for "idiopathic" pancreatitis?
2. When should you repeat imaging, and what modality should you use?
3. When is genetic testing appropriate?
4. What about autoimmune pancreatitis—when do you think of that?
5. Is empiric cholecystectomy ever warranted in idiopathic cases?
6. What is the role of ERCP or sphincter of Oddi evaluation in recurrent idiopathic AP?

Case 1.7: What do the guidelines say?

Source: ACG 2024 Acute Pancreatitis Guidelines[1]

Recurrent "idiopathic" pancreatitis is often idiopathic only because we quit looking too soon. The ACG guideline argues that a second—or certainly a third—flare without an identified cause should ignite a methodical, layered search rather than acceptance of mystery. Let's walk through that search, filling in the details behind each rung of the diagnostic ladder.

First Pass: Squeeze the Low-Hanging Fruit—*Twice*

Even excellent sonographers can miss grains of sludge when the duodenum is gas-packed or the patient can't hold a deep breath. For that reason, the guideline recommends repeating a RUQ ultrasound when the acute pain settles and the bowel is quieter. Tiny gallstones or dense "bouillabaisse" sludge (very descriptive...)—the most common hidden culprit—often declare themselves on the encore study. While you wait, be sure you have a complete metabolic screen: a fasting triglyceride panel (levels should top 1,000 mg/dL before they cause pancreatitis), an ionized or corrected calcium, and a hard look at the medication list for proven offenders such as azathioprine, 6-MP, valproate, hydrochlorothiazide, didanosine, or high-dose steroids. If any of those boxes remain blank, the case is not yet idiopathic.

> Recurrent unexplained pancreatitis? Make sure to:
> * Repeat U/S
> * Check fasting TG
> * Check ionized calcium
> * Look over meds

Escalating the View: EUS vs MRCP

When ultrasound, lipids, calcium, and drug audit are all clean, the guideline's next tier is high-resolution ductal imaging.

- Endoscopic ultrasound peers millimeters from the pancreatic head and hilum; it excels at catching microlithiasis, pancreas divisum, sub-centimeter tumors, and early chronic-pancreatitis changes that a CT misses.
- MRCP provides a panoramic, radiation-free map of the main duct and its side branches, beautifully demonstrating minor

anatomic variants and subtle strictures, especially when enhanced with secretin stimulation, while sparing the patient sedation.

The choice usually comes down to logistics: if you have an EUS-ERCP suite that can do a single-session "look, find, and treat," EUS first is elegant; otherwise, an MRCP that can be ordered from triage and performed within hours is perfectly guideline-sanctioned. **Figure 1.6** shows a MRCP showing classic pancreas divisum filling the dorsal duct.

Sidebar. Remember that pancreas divisum is a common anatomic variant—in up to 10% of the general population—but only a minority ever develop pancreatitis. Most studies suggest divisum alone is insufficient to cause attacks unless it coexists with another hit such as *CFTR* or *SPINK1* mutations. So, if you do find a divisum, interpret it in the full clinical and genetic context before calling it the smoking gun.

Figure 1.6. *Pancreas Divisum. MRCP showing the "crossing duct" sign where the common bile duct (a) crosses the larger dorsal duct of Santorini (b) draining through the minor papilla. Also, the smaller ventral duct of Wirsung (c) drains through the major papilla in pancreas divisum.*

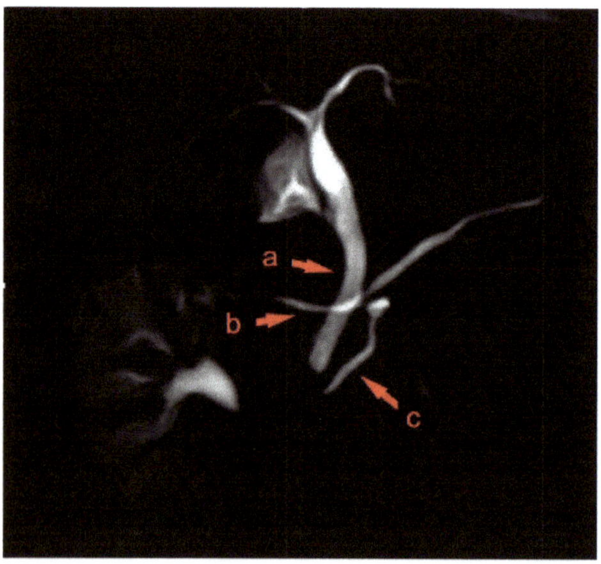

Metabolic and Immune Zebras

When EUS/MRCP still reveal no smoking gun, widen the net for autoimmune and genetic causes. A serum IgG4 can unmask type 1 autoimmune pancreatitis; an early trial of steroids is life-changing if the diagnosis is confirmed. Parallel to that, a focused 4-gene panel (*PRSS1, SPINK1, CFTR, CTRC*) is appropriate in young patients, those with 2 or more affected relatives, or anyone whose exhaustive anatomic workup is negative but attacks keep recurring. The yield is modest, yet a positive result guides counseling, informs family members, and in some cases, changes surveillance strategy.

Still no explanation after repeat U/S, TG, checking meds, MRCP or EUS for recurrent AP? Check IgG4 and genetic panel

Empiric Cholecystectomy

One of the most provocative ACG recommendations is empiric laparoscopic cholecystectomy after the second unexplained attack. A systematic review and meta-analysis showed that cholecystectomy after an episode of idiopathic acute pancreatitis (with negative EUS and MRCP) decreased the recurrence rate from 39% to 11%, presumably by clearing microlithiasis too small for any image to capture.[23] Laparoscopy is outpatient, low-risk, and, in fit patients, often easier than another spiral through the emergency department. If your surgeon is agreeable and the patient is surgically fit, the evidence supports getting the gallbladder out even when it looks perfectly innocent.

Consider empiric cholecystectomy for unexplained recurrent AP in surgically fit candidates

The Last Gate: ERCP with Manometry in Expert Hands

Only after repeat ultrasound, EUS or MRCP, autoimmune serology, genetics, and (ideally) cholecystectomy fail to stop the cycle does the guideline open the door to diagnostic ERCP. At that point you are searching for pancreatic sphincter of Oddi hypertension or a subtle divisum needing minor papilla therapy—scenarios that demand high-volume expertise, prophylactic pancreatic duct stenting, and immediate access to rescue care should PEP strike. Community centers should refer such patients to specialized pancreatology units.

Moreover, you really need to think twice about doing an ERCP in these patients since ERCP with sphincterotomy for suspected sphincter of Oddi dysfunction did not reduce disability due to pain in a randomized trial.[24]

See **Table 1.5** for a summary of steps for diagnosing unexplained recurrent AP.

Table 1.5 *Steps for Diagnosing Unexplained Recurrent AP.*

Step	Key tool / action	Typical yield
1	Repeat RUQ ultrasound; fasting TG; corrected Ca; drug audit	Microlithiasis, hyper-TG, hyper-Ca, culprit drugs
2	EUS or MRCP	Divisum, micro-stones, early neoplasm, duct strictures
3	IgG4, then 4-gene panel (*PRSS1, SPINK1, CFTR, CTRC*) when criteria met	Autoimmune pancreatitis; hereditary variants
4	Empiric laparoscopic cholecystectomy after ≥2 unexplained attacks	Eliminates occult biliary microlithiasis; cuts recurrence
5	ERCP ± manometry only in expert centers	SOD type 2, therapy for divisum

Now, let's apply these diagnostic principles to the case. Our 40-year-old "mystery man" has never had the second-look ultrasound, an EUS, or an MRCP, and no one has checked his IgG4 or family pedigree. You should arrange the missing imaging before discharge, draw autoimmune panels, discuss genetics given his young age, and schedule surgical clinic in case the next round is still blank. Only if every step remains negative, and attacks continue, will you consider sending him to a tertiary center for sphincter manometry and possible pancreatic sphincterotomy.

Bottom line: "Idiopathic" is a diagnosis of persistence, not resignation. Climb the entire ladder and most mysteries reveal the culprit before you reach the top.

Case 1.8: No Stones, Still Groans

A 45-year-old man presents to your clinic with a 5-year history of recurrent upper abdominal pain. The pain is postprandial, dull and crampy, centered in the epigastrium, and sometimes radiates to the back. He describes "flare-ups" that occur every few weeks, often lasting several days. He's lost about 15 pounds over the past year due to fear of eating and has been told at various times that he has "IBS," "gastritis," and "functional dyspepsia."

He does not drink alcohol and has no history of gallstones, smoking, or trauma. Family history is non-contributory.

Labs show a normal CBC, metabolic panel, HbA1c, and lipase. Fecal elastase is borderline at 200 µg/g. Abdominal ultrasound is unremarkable. A contrast-enhanced CT scan done last year during a pain flare showed no pancreatic calcifications or ductal changes.

He's frustrated and exhausted. *I don't want narcotics*, he says. *But I want an answer.* He asks you directly: *Could this still be my pancreas, even though all the scans are normal*?

Know your guidelines!

1. How is chronic pancreatitis defined in the modern ACG guideline?
2. What imaging and functional tests are appropriate when chronic pancreatitis is suspected but CT and ultrasound are normal?
3. When should you consider autoimmune pancreatitis, genetic testing, or early CP in low-risk patients?
4. What's the role of EUS and endoscopic function testing in "minimal change" disease?
5. How do we avoid both over-diagnosis and under-diagnosis in patients with chronic upper abdominal pain?

Case 1.8: What do the guidelines say?

Source: ACG 2020 Chronic Pancreatitis Guidelines[25]

The frustration here is palpable—and justified. This patient has classic symptoms of chronic pancreatitis (CP): upper abdominal pain, postprandial flares, weight loss from fear of eating, and a gradual decline in quality of life. And yet, his labs are unremarkable, his imaging is clean, and he's been bounced around with vague diagnoses like IBS and functional dyspepsia. The question is fair: *Could this still be his pancreas, even with normal tests*? According to the ACG guideline by Gardner et al., the answer is **yes!**

A New Way of Thinking About CP

We've come a long way from defining chronic pancreatitis as calcifications and duct dilation on CT. The latest guidelines adopt a mechanistic definition: chronic pancreatitis is a fibro-inflammatory syndrome of the pancreas, characterized by progressive damage to parenchyma and ducts, leading to chronic pain, exocrine and endocrine dysfunction, and a wide range of complications. In this model, imaging findings can lag behind pathophysiology, and diagnosis depends on a combination of clinical suspicion, imaging, functional testing, and risk factors

> Remember that imaging findings can lag behind pathophysiology and clinical course in CP

So yes, this patient may have early or "minimal change" chronic pancreatitis. The job now is to move past the normal CT and dig deeper.

When First-Line Imaging Is Normal, What Comes Next?

The guideline recommends a stepwise diagnostic approach. This patient has already had a normal abdominal ultrasound and a contrast-enhanced CT—both are appropriate first-line tests. But when these are unrevealing and clinical suspicion remains high, EUS is the next test of choice.[26] EUS can detect subtle parenchymal changes, such as hyperechoic foci, stranding, and ductal irregularity—findings that may support early CP in the right clinical setting.

If EUS is non-diagnostic, but suspicion for CP remains high—due to typical symptoms, borderline fecal elastase, and unexplained weight loss—the guideline suggests advancing to secretin-enhanced MRCP (s-MRCP). This test allows non-invasive visualization of ductal anatomy and, crucially, gives a functional readout of exocrine pancreatic secretion by assessing duodenal filling after secretin stimulation.[27] In minimal change disease, this can be the deciding factor that tips you toward—or away from—a diagnosis.

If you suspect CP but CT is negative, do EUS next. If negative, consider s-MRCP

Importantly, direct pancreatic function testing via endoscopy (i.e., collecting duodenal fluid and measuring bicarbonate levels) is not recommended by the ACG guideline as part of the routine diagnostic workup for CP. Its use is complementary and largely reserved for evaluating exocrine pancreatic insufficiency (EPI), rather than establishing the diagnosis of CP itself.

What Else Should We Be Thinking About?

The guideline emphasizes the importance of broadening your lens, especially in younger or low-risk patients. Our patient doesn't drink alcohol, doesn't smoke, and has no clear mechanical risk factors. This is exactly the scenario where autoimmune and genetic causes should be considered.

- ***Autoimmune pancreatitis*** (AIP) may present with subtle or non-specific findings. In type 1 AIP, look for elevated serum IgG4 levels and extrapancreatic manifestations (e.g., salivary gland swelling, biliary strictures). Type 2 AIP is harder to pin down serologically and often requires histology or response to steroids.
- ***Genetic testing*** is appropriate when patients are young (typically <35–40), have a family history of pancreatitis, or are considered idiopathic after initial workup. The guideline suggests testing for *PRSS1, SPINK1, CFTR*, and *CTRC* mutations. In some cases, the combination of genetic risk factors and environmental modifiers (e.g., smoking, dietary factors) can tip the scale toward disease progression.

How Do We Avoid Over-Diagnosis in Chronic Upper Abdominal Pain?

This is where clinical wisdom matters. Not every case of epigastric discomfort is chronic pancreatitis, and the guideline warns against labeling patients prematurely—especially in the absence of risk factors, imaging changes, or objective exocrine/endocrine dysfunction. Red flags that increase your pretest probability of CP might include:

- Typical postprandial pain that radiates to the back
- Recurrent flares over months or years
- Documented weight loss
- Borderline or low fecal elastase (like our patient's 200 μg/g)
- Known risk factors (e.g., alcohol, smoking, genetic mutations)

On the other hand, bloating, gas, and diffuse abdominal pain without a pattern—especially in patients with psychiatric comorbidities or a strong IBS history—should raise your threshold for diagnosing CP because they tend to argue against a pancreatic source, although everyone is different. The guideline doesn't give a score or formula. It gives you tools—and trusts you to interpret them in context.

Bringing It Together

This patient may very well have early chronic pancreatitis, even though his scans are normal. The next steps include:

1. EUS to assess subtle parenchymal and ductal features
2. If equivocal, consider s-MRCP
3. Check IgG4 and evaluate for autoimmune features
4. Consider genetic testing given the absence of risk factors and his age
5. Avoid the temptation to diagnose based on symptoms alone—but don't dismiss the pancreas just because the CT was clean

He doesn't want narcotics—he wants an explanation. And the guidelines give you a clear, stepwise approach to help get him there.

Let's get him scheduled for EUS.

Case 1.9: Echoes Without Certainty

Your 45-year-old patient with recurrent upper abdominal pain and weight loss undergoes EUS to evaluate for CP. His prior CT and abdominal ultrasound were normal, but his clinical picture raised concern for early or "minimal change" CP. He has no history of alcohol use, smoking, gallstones, or known genetic risk factors.

The EUS report notes 3 parenchymal features (lobularity, echogenic foci, and hyperechoic strands) and 1 ductal feature (main duct irregularity), all described as "mild." There are no calcifications, no cysts or masses, and no obvious ductal dilation. The endoscopist concludes: "Findings suggestive but not diagnostic of early chronic pancreatitis. Clinical correlation advised."

Your patient wants answers. *Does this mean I have it?* he asks. *And if this doesn't prove anything, what do we do now?*

Know your guidelines!

1. What is the diagnostic value of EUS in CP?
2. How are EUS findings interpreted, and what criteria increase specificity?
3. What is the Rosemont classification?
4. If the EUS is equivocal, what's the next best test?
5. How do we counsel patients when findings are indeterminate?

Case 1.9: What do the guidelines say?

Source: ACG 2020 Chronic Pancreatitis Guidelines[24]

This is the EUS report that makes everyone squirm: a few findings, nothing definitive, and the dreaded phrase "clinical correlation advised." You're left wondering whether to stamp "early CP" on the chart or admit that, after all that workup, you're still in diagnostic limbo. According to the ACG guideline, this is precisely the kind of scenario that demands both restraint and precision.

What Do We Do With a Borderline EUS?

First, let's remind ourselves: EUS is a highly sensitive tool, but it's not terribly specific. It picks up subtle parenchymal and ductal changes that other modalities can miss—but many of those changes also occur in aging, smoking, diabetes, obesity, and even in healthy individuals. So, the key is not just how many features are present, but also which ones, and in what context.

EUS is sensitive, but not specific, for early CP

In this case, the EUS showed 3 parenchymal features (lobularity, echogenic foci, and strands) and 1 ductal feature (main duct irregularity)—which meets the commonly used threshold of 4 or more features that may suggest CP. **Figure 1.7** shows some EUS findings of subtle CP.

Figure 1.7. *EUS features of CP, (left) parenchymal lobularity, stranding and echogenic foci and (right) irregular main pancreatic duct with hyperechoic duct wall.*[28]

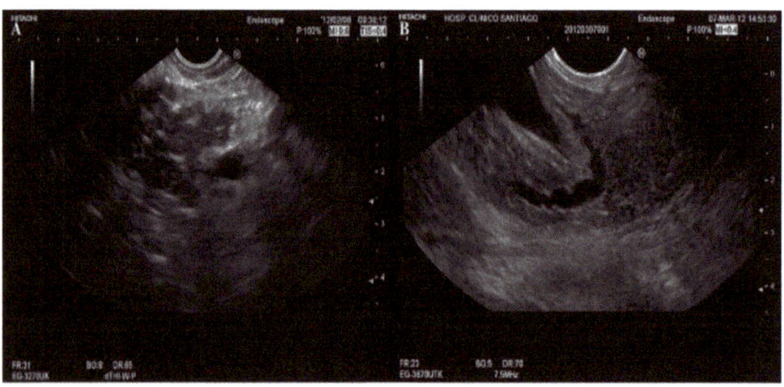

But the guideline emphasizes that EUS findings alone are not sufficient to make the diagnosis of chronic pancreatitis—especially when they are mild and not accompanied by clinical or functional evidence of pancreatic insufficiency or progressive damage. So, how do we proceed with this case?

EUS findings alone are insufficient to definitively diagnose CP

You might be tempted to pull out the **Rosemont classification**—a system that categorizes EUS findings into "consistent with," "suggestive of," or "indeterminate for" chronic pancreatitis based on a weighted scoring scheme.[29] While this framework has historical value, the ACG CP guideline neither endorses nor emphasizes its use. In fact, it cautions against relying on a limited number of EUS features to make the diagnosis in isolation. As noted earlier, many of the parenchymal and ductal abnormalities detected on EUS can also appear in aging, smoking, diabetes, or even healthy individuals. Rather than leaning on a rigid scoring system, the guideline favors a more practical approach—one that integrates EUS findings with clinical suspicion, risk factors, and, when needed, complementary testing like s-MRCP or evaluation for exocrine insufficiency.

If the Rosemont classification doesn't get us there, where does that leave us? This EUS result doesn't close the case—it keeps it open. The next recommended step, per the guideline, is to obtain an s-MRCP, as mentioned in the last vignette. This test serves 2 purposes: it provides high-quality ductal imaging and assesses pancreatic exocrine function by visualizing duodenal fluid filling after secretin stimulation. A lack of duodenal filling or delayed flow can suggest early ductal dysfunction, which may support the diagnosis of early CP in the right clinical context.

As mentioned in the last vignette, the guideline makes clear that direct pancreatic function testing—i.e., collecting duodenal fluid via endoscopy to measure bicarbonate—is complementary, but not routinely required in the diagnostic workup of CP. It's more commonly used when evaluating for exocrine pancreatic insufficiency rather than establishing a diagnosis of CP itself.

How Do We Talk to the Patient?

You don't have a slam dunk diagnosis yet—and that's okay. The guideline supports taking a cautious, data-driven approach when imaging findings are borderline. Your explaination to the patient can be something like:

These results suggest there might be early changes in your pancreas, but they're not definitive. The next step is a more specialized MRI that can help us see how your pancreas is functioning in real time. That will give us a better sense of whether your symptoms are related to early pancreatitis or something else.

This language helps the patient feel heard—while reinforcing that you're not guessing or labeling prematurely.

Bottom line: In patients with high clinical suspicion but non-diagnostic CT or MRI, EUS is the next best test. But when EUS reveals only mild or equivocal findings, the ACG guideline recommends proceeding to s-MRCP to assess for functional abnormalities. Diagnosis of CP should ideally not rest on EUS alone—especially when the findings are subtle.

This case underscores a central theme in the modern approach to chronic pancreatitis: we're not chasing checkboxes—we're integrating data, context, and caution. That's how we move from noise to clarity. And for this patient, it means 1 more test—not an answer yet, but a smarter question.

Case 1.10: Now What?

Your 45-year-old patient with chronic postprandial epigastric pain, weight loss, and prior non-diagnostic CT and borderline EUS findings has just completed his s-MRCP. This test finally offers some clarity: delayed enhancement after contrast and irregularity of the main pancreatic duct, consistent with CP (**Figure 1.8**).

Figure 1.8. *Results of s-MRCP.*[30]

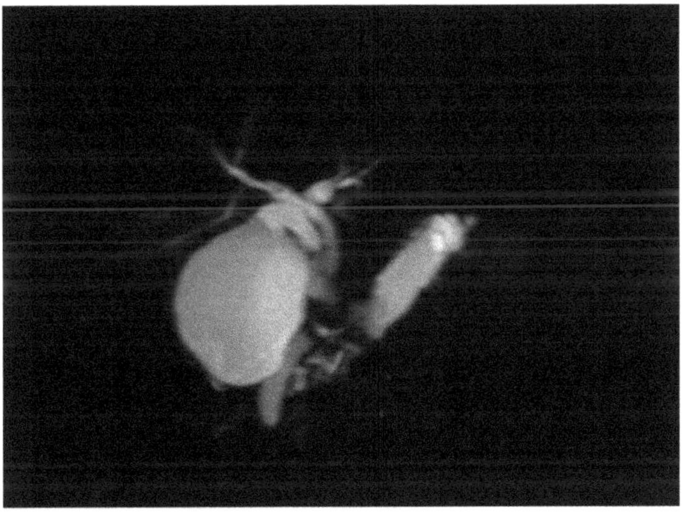

Know your guidelines!

1. Once CP is diagnosed, how do we determine why it happened?
2. What is the TIGAR-O framework and how is it used?
3. When should we consider genetic testing or evaluation for AIP?
4. What are the first steps in managing early CP?
5. When should pancreatic enzyme therapy be started?
6. What labs and clinical parameters should be monitored over time?

Case 1.10: What do the guidelines say?

Source: ACG 2020 Chronic Pancreatitis Guidelines[25]

This is the pivot point. After years of pain, weight loss, and normal imaging, your patient finally has a diagnosis: CP, confirmed by s-MRCP. The fog is starting to clear—but he's right to ask: *what now*?

The ACG guideline helps you build a smart, personalized plan from here. That starts with answering two questions: What caused it? And what can we do to slow it down, manage symptoms, and prevent complications?

Step 1: Identify the cause—or at least rule out the big ones

The guideline's diagnostic framework begins with TIGAR-O, a helpful mnemonic that classifies etiologies by mechanism. **Table 1.6** lays out the TIGAR-O components for diagnosing CP.

Table. 1.6. *TIGAR-O Diagnoses for CP.*

TIGAR-O Category	Examples
Toxic-metabolic	Alcohol, tobacco, hypercalcemia, hypertriglyceridemia, chronic renal failure, medications
Idiopathic	No identifiable cause (often early-onset or "minimal change" disease)
Genetic	*PRSS1, SPINK1, CFTR, CTRC* mutations
Autoimmune	Type 1 AIP (IgG4-related), Type 2 AIP
Recurrent acute	Especially post-ERCP, trauma, or viral infections
Obstructive	Pancreas divisum, ductal stricture, tumors, ampullary stenosis

This patient has no history of alcohol, smoking, trauma, or gallstones, and he's only 45—so you're in idiopathic territory for now. But the guideline warns not to accept that label too quickly. In cases like this, where clinical suspicion is high and no clear etiology has emerged, it's time to consider testing for autoimmune and genetic causes.

- Check serum IgG4. Type 1 autoimmune pancreatitis can be subtle at onset and may present without biliary involvement. Even a mildly elevated IgG4 can warrant further workup or an empiric trial of steroids.
- Genetic testing is appropriate here. The guideline recommends considering *PRSS1, SPINK1, CFTR*, and *CTRC* testing in patients with idiopathic CP, especially if early-onset or there's a family history of pancreatitis, cystic fibrosis, or pancreatic cancer. Genetic counseling is ideal if available—but shouldn't be a barrier to testing if access is limited.

Step 2: Focus early management on function—not just pain

The cornerstone of CP management is preserving pancreatic function, especially early in the disease course and preventing progression—not just treating flares. That starts with a few immediate priorities.

Nutrition. Patients with CP are at risk for malnutrition, vitamin deficiencies, and low bone density. He's already lost 15 pounds. The guideline recommends checking:

- Fecal elastase (already done, borderline at 200)
- Fat-soluble vitamins (A, D, E, K)
- Prealbumin and zinc
- Bone density (DEXA scan) if weight loss, malabsorption, or long-standing disease

Exocrine pancreatic insufficiency (EPI). His fecal elastase is borderline—but what does that really mean? Fecal elastase-1 is a noninvasive marker of exocrine pancreatic function, specifically testing the concentration of elastase in the stool. Because elastase is secreted by the pancreas and remains stable during intestinal transit, it gives a reliable snapshot of how much digestive enzyme output is reaching the gut. Levels are interpreted as follows:

- >200 μg/g = normal
- 100–200 μg/g = borderline or mild EPI
- <100 μg/g = severe EPI

The test is most helpful in patients with chronic symptoms of

Borderline elastase in suspected CP? Consider PERT

malabsorption—weight loss, steatorrhea, bloating, or fat-soluble vitamin deficiency. However, like many tests, it's not perfect. Borderline values like his (200 μg/g) live in a gray zone: not normal, but not clearly diagnostic either. In these cases, the guideline supports a clinical trial of pancreatic enzyme replacement therapy (PERT)—especially if symptoms suggest maldigestion. More on PERT soon.

Elastase is less sensitive in early CP and can be inccurate

It's worth noting that fecal elastase is less sensitive in early disease, and results can be falsely normal in patients with rapid transit time in diarrhea with less enzyme degradation. Moreover, results can be falsely abnormal in patients with watery diarrhea or loose stool, which dilutes the sample. So, it should not be the sole deciding factor. As always, treat the patient, not the number—but the number helps shape the decision.

Endocrine function. CP increases risk for Type 3c diabetes—pancreatogenic diabetes, which is often brittle and insulin-dependent. His HbA1c is normal now, but should be checked annually moving forward.

Step 3: What about pain?

PERT is not a primary treatment for abdominal pain

The ACG is clear here: PERT is not a primary pain treatment in early CP (although PERT is useful for symptoms of EPI). For mild-to-moderate pain, begin with supportive strategies, including:

Remind patients to remain abstinent from alcohol and smoking, even if prior exposure was minimal. You also might consider antioxidant supplements to treat pain in CP

- Eat smaller, more frequent meals
- Avoid high-fat loads that trigger postprandial pain
- Remain abstinent from alcohol and smoking even if prior exposure was minimal—both are risk factors for progression
- Consider antioxidant supplements (e.g., selenium, vitamin C/E, methionine), especially in early disease. The guideline gives this a conditional recommendation—it's no panacea, but low-risk and possibly helpful.

Pain escalations should not be managed with narcotics alone, especially early in the disease course. If pain persists or worsens, imaging (EUS or MRCP) should be repeated to assess for obstructive complications (e.g., dominant duct stricture, stones, pseudocyst), and referred to a pancreatology center for possible endoscopic or surgical intervention. Of note, referral would be appropriate for this patient – look again at that MRCP, which showed some stones in the distal portion of the main pancreatic duct.

Step 4: Set the pace for long-term follow-up

CP is a chronic condition, not a 1-stop shop. This is the moment to build a relationship and lay out a monitoring plan:

- Annual labs: HbA1c, vitamin levels, nutritional markers
- Repeat fecal elastase every 6-12 months or if symptoms change
- DEXA scan every 2-3 years
- Monitor weight, bowel habits, and quality of life at each visit
- If a genetic mutation is found, additional counseling and family screening may be appropriate. If autoimmune markers are positive, consider GI or rheumatology referral to assess for systemic involvement.

Bringing It Together

This is CP—and early is the best time to catch it. You've now confirmed the diagnosis with s-MRCP, and the next steps are clear: search for the etiology, protect glandular function, and manage pain carefully without overtreating it with narcotics if at all possible. This is also the moment to start building a long-term plan and clinical partnership. The patient has waited years for someone to take this seriously—now he's got the diagnosis, and with it, a clear path forward.

Case 1.11: The Pain That Won't Quit

Six months have passed since your 45-year-old patient was initially diagnosed with CP, confirmed by s-MRCP. You completed an etiology workup—no alcohol, no smoking, normal IgG4, and a negative genetic panel. He's been adherent to PERT, avoids alcohol, eats a low-fat diet, and his vitamin levels and weight have stabilized.

But the pain hasn't.

He describes a deep, dull ache in his epigastrium, worse after eating, and radiating to the back. It flares up several times a week and sometimes wakes him from sleep. His quality of life has cratered—he's missing work, sleeping poorly, and increasingly anxious. His primary care physician started him on low-dose hydrocodone 2 months ago, and he now finds himself needing it more frequently to get through the day.

A repeat CT shows a dilated pancreatic duct measuring 7 mm, and now without calcifications or visible stones. His enzymes and blood work are stable, and he remains on high-dose pancreatic enzymes and acid suppression with a proton pump inhibitor (PPI).

Know your guidelines!

1. What's the recommended stepwise approach to pain in CP?
2. When are opioids appropriate?
3. Does PERT help with pain? (hint: no!)
4. What's the role of endoscopic therapy or surgery in ductal disease?
5. When should you consider celiac plexus block or TPIAT?
6. How do we match the intervention to the anatomy?

Case 1.11: What do the guidelines say?

Source: ACG 2020 Chronic Pancreatitis Guidelines[25]

This is where managing CP shifts from algorithm to art. Our patient has done everything right: no alcohol, no smoking, compliant with enzyme therapy, and eating carefully. His weight has stabilized, his labs look fine, and he's on acid suppression to optimize PERT delivery. But despite all that, the pain marches on. These are among the toughest CP cases a gastroenterologist can manage.

The ACG guideline recognizes this challenge: pain is the most common symptom in CP, but it's also the most complex to manage. Unlike exocrine or endocrine dysfunction, which you can track with lab values and adjust with dosing, pain in CP is multifactorial, often poorly correlated with imaging, and notoriously difficult to treat. That said, the guideline gives us a clear, structured path to follow to give our patients the best shot.

> Pancreatic enzymes are inactivated by acid, so adding a PPI can help optimize PERT

Check Your Foundation

The first step is to confirm the basics are optimized. He's already on high-dose pancreatic enzymes and a proton pump inhibitor (PPI)—and that combination matters. Pancreatic enzymes are inactivated by gastric acid, so adding a PPI can help protect the enzymes from acid degradation, especially in patients who don't fully respond to PERT alone. The guideline notes that acid suppression may improve enzyme effectiveness, particularly in patients with persistent symptoms despite appropriate dosing. But just to be clear: PERT is not a primary pain medication. The idea that enzymes "rest the pancreas" and reduce pain comes from older theories. The ACG guideline states plainly that enzyme therapy should not be used to treat pain unless exocrine insufficiency is present. In this case, PERT is being used appropriately—for borderline elastase and weight loss—not for pain relief. The PPI is there to make that enzyme therapy work better—not to solve the pain on its own.

> Once again, don't use PERT other than to manage pain. Use it for exocrine insufficiency

PD numbers to know:

* ≤2 mm in body/tail is normal
* ≤3 mm in head is normal
* ≥5 mm is abnormal

It's also worth rechecking that no reversible anatomic process is being missed. His CT shows a 7 mm pancreatic duct, which meets criteria for ductal dilation. In general, the normal main pancreatic duct is ≤3 mm in the head and ≤ 2 mm in the body and tail. Anything ≥5 mm is often considered abnormal, and ≥6 mm is typically used as the threshold for "large duct" disease in CP. A 7 mm duct puts him solidly in that category.

While there are no visible stones or strictures, cross-sectional imaging can miss small obstructing lesions or a dominant stricture near the head of the pancreas. That's why MRCP or EUS—if not recently done—are still worth pursuing, to exclude a subtle obstruction that may be amenable to drainage. If a mechanical issue is found—like a tight stricture or an impacted stone—that opens the door to endoscopic or surgical decompression, which the guideline supports as a pain-relieving intervention in patients with large duct disease. In other words, this is the moment to double-check whether there's a target before we escalate therapy.

If Anatomy's Clear, Escalate Gradually

Once you've ruled out a fixable lesion, and the enzymes and acid suppression are optimized, the guideline recommends a step-up approach to pain. This begins with supportive strategies that we discussed in the last vignette: small, frequent meals; alcohol and smoking abstinence (check, check); and in early disease, a trial of antioxidant therapy. The data here are mixed, but antioxidants like vitamin C, vitamin E, selenium, and methionine may help reduce oxidative stress on pancreatic nerves. They won't work for everyone, but the downside is minimal, and some patients experience real relief.[31]

Benefits outweigh risks of antioxidant therapy for CP pain

If the pain persists despite these measures—and especially if it's interfering with function—it's time to look deeper at anatomy. This patient has a dilated duct, which places him in the subset where endoscopic or surgical decompression may be appropriate. The guideline highlights that for patients with large duct disease (typically duct ≥ 6 mm), endoscopic therapy—such as pancreatic sphincterotomy, ductal stenting, or stone clearance—can provide relief. The response may not be permanent, and re-intervention is common, but for many, it's enough to change the trajectory.

Interestingly, the guideline also points out that surgical drainage (e.g., Puestow procedure) may be superior to endoscopic treatment in terms of long-term pain relief, based on randomized trials. That said, it's rarely first-line and is typically reserved for patients with failed endoscopic therapy or anatomic considerations that make surgery more favorable. This is where shared decision-making, surgical referral, and ideally care at a center with pancreatology expertise become key.

What About Opioids?

Let's talk about the medication creeping into his routine. The guideline is blunt: opioids should not be the foundation of pain management in CP. They may be necessary for some patients, especially in the short-term, but they should always be a last resort—used only after supportive, nutritional, and procedural strategies have been exhausted. Chronic opioid use comes with well-known baggage: tolerance, dependence, hyperalgesia, and in some cases, worsening of the central pain phenotype. If opioids are used, they should be carefully titrated, monitored, and ideally co-managed with pain specialists. Also, if you're going down this road, be sure to consider sending the patient for cognitive behavioral therapy (CBT) which has demonstrated benefits for helping to manage CP pain.

Consider CBT as non-pharmacological adjunctive therapy for CP pain

A quick aside on advanced options. For patients with intractable pain, even after endoscopic or surgical therapy, celiac plexus block may be considered. It's more commonly used in malignancy-related pain, but in selected cases of CP, particularly with central sensitization, it may offer temporary benefit.[32]

In rare, severe, refractory cases—especially in patients with early-onset disease, genetic mutations, or brittle diabetes—the ultimate intervention is total pancreatectomy with islet autotransplantation (TPIAT).[33] This is a massive step, requiring specialized evaluation, and is typically reserved for young patients with disabling pain, minimal morphologic change, and no ongoing substance use.

Bringing It Home

Your patient has reached the "now what?" stage. His duct is dilated. His enzymes and acid suppression are already optimized. He's on escalating narcotics—and he's still miserable. Per the ACG guideline, this is the perfect time to:

- Confirm anatomy with MRCP or EUS
- Refer to advanced endoscopy for possible ductal decompression
- Consider a trial of antioxidants
- Start a conversation with a pancreatobiliary surgeon if endoscopy fails
- Loop in a pain specialist if opioids remain necessary

There's no quick fix—but there is a path forward. And more importantly, he's no longer on it alone with multidisciplinary support.

Case 1.12: Mustard Sausage Signal

You're asked to weigh in on a 66-year-old man admitted for painless jaundice. He was at Wrigley Field watching his beloved Chicago Cubs and noted that his eyes looked like the color of mustard on his sausage at the ballpark. Thus, he became alarmed and came in for evaluation. His labs show a total bilirubin of 4.9 mg/dL and an ALP of 590. AST and ALT are modestly elevated, and lipase is normal. A CT scan done in the emergency department shows a diffusely enlarged pancreas with loss of normal lobularity, a narrowed distal common bile duct, and mild intrahepatic biliary dilation. There's no discrete mass.

His history is notable for a prior diagnosis of "chronic pancreatitis" 8 years ago, made after recurrent bouts of abdominal pain and some pancreatic "fullness" on a prior CT. He rarely drinks, doesn't smoke, and has no family history of pancreatic cancer. He's had no surgeries, no inflammatory bowel disease (IBD), and no recent travel.

On review of systems, he reports recent fatigue, a 10-pound weight loss over the last 6 weeks, and a dry mouth, which he hadn't mentioned before. No fever, night sweats, or diarrhea.

Labs today show: IgG4 is normal; CA 19-9 is 62 U/mL; total IgG is elevated at 2100 mg/dL; ANA is positive at 1:160; amylase and lipase are normal. A CT scan from 9 years ago notes a "prominent pancreas" but no calcifications or ductal dilation.

GI is consulted for concern for pancreatic cancer vs chronic pancreatitis. The radiologist isn't convinced it's a tumor—but they're not ruling it out either.

Know your guidelines!

1. When should you suspect AIP, and how does it differ from classic CP or pancreatic cancer?
2. What are the distinguishing features of type 1 vs type 2 AIP?
3. How sensitive and specific is serum IgG4 testing?

4. What are the hallmark imaging features of AIP?
5. When is it appropriate to offer a trial of steroids, and how should you monitor response?
6. How often is AIP misdiagnosed as CP—and when should you reconsider the original diagnosis?

Case 1.12: What do the guidelines say?

Source: ACG 2020 Chronic Pancreatitis Guidelines[25]

It's easy to see how this patient landed in diagnostic purgatory. He has painless jaundice, a diffusely enlarged pancreas, and vague systemic symptoms—plus a past label of "chronic pancreatitis" that's been sitting in his chart for almost a decade. The radiologist isn't calling it cancer, but they're not ruling it out either. It smells like CP, but doesn't behave like it. The CT shows fullness, not atrophy; no calcifications, no chain of lakes duct, and no sign of a clear-cut mass, although one never knows when it comes to the pancreas.

It's time to press pause and consider the great pancreatic tumor imitator: AIP.

The ACG guideline calls AIP a distinct, often reversible subtype of CP, and reminds us that missing it can lead to unnecessary stents, surgery, and even pancreatectomy. So, when do you suspect it? The clues are all over this case: older age at onset, painless jaundice, imaging showing a "plump" pancreas rather than a scarred one, and extra hints like elevated total IgG and a positive ANA. The cherry on top? A previous diagnosis of CP that never really fit.

Type 1 vs Type 2: Know the Difference

Typically, Type 1 AIP is part of IgG4-related disease; whereas, Type 2 AIP is more often seen in younger patients with IBD.

Type I AIP: Part of IgG4-related disease

Type II AIP: Often seen in younger patients with IBD

This patient fits the **Type 1** mold: older age, male, vague constitutional symptoms, and possible salivary gland involvement (remember the dry mouth?). Type 1 AIP can involve nearly any organ—the bile ducts, kidneys, retroperitoneum, lungs—and is associated with elevated serum IgG4 levels in about 70% of cases. But here's the kicker: a normal IgG4 doesn't rule it out. That's why it's important to check the total IgG, ANA, and imaging as additional diagnostic support. He checks all of those boxes.

Remember that a normal IgG4 doesn't rule out Type 1 AIP

Type 2 AIP, by contrast, is seronegative, doesn't involve other organs, and often requires histology for diagnosis. It's more commonly found in younger individuals with ulcerative colitis or Crohn's disease and tends to respond briskly to steroids. But that's not your guy here.

Imaging Holds the Key

Classic imaging features of both Type 1 and Type 2 AIP include a "sausage-shaped" pancreas—enlarged, featureless, and hypodense—along with a capsule-like rim and narrowed main pancreatic duct. This is a major branch point in the diagnostic algorithm. Unlike CP, where the duct is typically dilated and irregular, AIP shows a long, smooth narrowing without upstream dilation. And rather than atrophy, the gland is enlarged and homogenous—like someone inflated it. Your patient's CT already hinted at that, but MRI with MRCP is often more telling. When you get the scan, it confirms it: a sausage-shaped pancreas, smooth delayed enhancement, and a narrowed but non-obstructed duct. **Figure 1.9** illustrates this classic appearance.

> Classic imaging features of AIP:
> * Sausage-shaped pancreas
> * Capsule-like rim or "halo"
> * Thin, attenuated main PD

Figure 1.9. *Autoimmune Pancreatitis. Note the diffuse enlargement or "sausage-shaped" pancreas, capsule-like rim, and thin main pancreatic duct on CT scan. There is no sign of a discrete mass, arguing against primary pancreatic cancer.*[34]

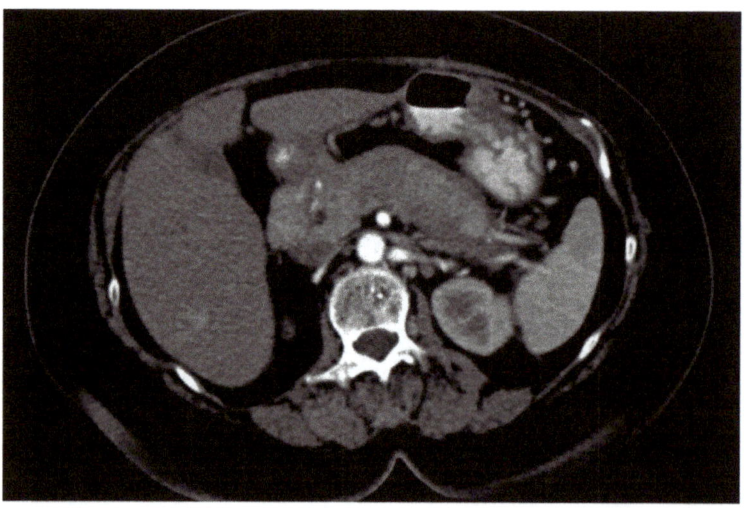

What About Biopsy?

Well, biopsy isn't always required—especially when imaging, serologies, and extrapancreatic clues align. In this case, you already have 3 pieces: imaging, serology (elevated total IgG, ANA), and extrapancreatic symptoms. If you were still uncertain, EUS-guided biopsy using a core needle could help. But it's reasonable here to proceed directly to a diagnostic trial of corticosteroids.

The Steroid Trial: How and Why

The guideline supports a short course of steroids (e.g., prednisone 30-40 mg/day) as a diagnostic and therapeutic tool in suspected AIP. Most patients respond dramatically—jaundice resolves, pain disappears, weight returns, and the pancreas visibly shrinks on repeat imaging within 2-4 weeks. That's your confirmation. If he improves, you taper the steroids over 8-12 weeks, and consider low-dose maintenance in high-risk patients or those with frequent relapse.

> Suspect AIP? Consider a short course of steroids. This can often be done before biopsy to rule out cancer, but use your judgment

Just as important: if he doesn't improve, the workup for pancreatic cancer resumes. That's why you always obtain baseline imaging and serologies before steroids, and follow the response closely. The ACG doesn't mandate biopsy or steroid trial first—it lets the clinical picture guide your choice.

Bringing It Together

This case isn't cancer. And it's not classic calcific CP. It's likely Type 1 AIP, and the ACG guideline gives you a path forward: recognize the clues, confirm with imaging, and use a carefully monitored trial of steroids to clinch the diagnosis. His past diagnosis of CP may have been an early form of AIP that smoldered quietly for years. Now the disease is active—and treatable. The patient is happy too since he can get back to the ballpark to root for the Cubbies!

> The Chicago Cubs finally got that elusive World Series title in 2016 and hope for many more!

Autoimmune pancreatitis is a great reminder that not all pancreatic disease is progressive. Sometimes, the pancreas just wants a little prednisone.

Case 1.13: Incidental Cyst

A 63-year-old woman is referred to you after a 2.4-cm pancreatic cyst was found on an abdominal CT done for flank pain and suspected nephrolithiasis. Her pain resolved quickly, and a Kidney, Ureter, and Bladder (KUB) X-ray confirmed a passed stone. She feels fine now, has no abdominal symptoms, and has no history of pancreatitis, trauma, jaundice, or GI complaints.

She has never smoked, drinks socially, and has no family history of pancreatic cancer. She does recall a bout of "really bad food poisoning" 5 years ago that landed her in the ED, but doesn't remember whether she had imaging at the time.

The CT report describes a well-circumscribed, unilocular cyst in the pancreatic tail measuring 2.4 cm, with no solid component or obvious communication with the pancreatic duct. No mural nodules or calcifications are noted. The main pancreatic duct appears normal in caliber.

Know your guidelines!

1. What are the most common types of pancreatic cysts, and how do we distinguish them on imaging?
2. What features define a worrisome cyst?
3. When is EUS and/or FNA appropriate?
4. What is the role of CEA, amylase, and cytology in cyst fluid?
5. How often should this cyst be surveilled?
6. When is surgery indicated?

Case 1.13: What do the guidelines say?

Source: ACG 2018 Pancreatic Cyst Guidelines[35]

This is one of the most common consults in outpatient GI: An incidental pancreatic cyst, found while someone was looking for something else. It's easy for patients—and sometimes their doctors—to assume the worst. But the ACG guidelines make a point of emphasizing that the vast majority of pancreatic cysts are benign or low-risk, and very few ever turn into cancer. The challenge is knowing which ones can be left alone, which need surveillance, and which deserve a closer look.

In this case, the patient is a 63-year-old woman with a 2.4-cm unilocular cyst in the pancreatic tail, discovered during a CT scan for kidney stones. She's asymptomatic, has no history of pancreatitis, and the CT describes no mural nodule, no thickened wall, no calcifications, and a normal pancreatic duct. It was found by accident, does not appear to be clearly dangerous, and is sitting in that in-between space where being aggressive could lead to unnecessary procedures, but being lax could, in the worst-case scenario, lead to a missed cancer. So, you gotta know your guidelines to keep things straight! Let's walk through the steps.

Step 1: What kind of cyst is it?

The ACG guidelines don't require you to label the cyst with 100% certainty, but it helps to build a differential based on context. Age, gender, location, and imaging clues narrow the list. Here, the patient is a woman in her 60s with a cyst in the tail, no history of pancreatitis, and no ductal connection seen on CT. That narrows the field:

- A serous cystadenoma (SCA) is less likely as they are typically microcystic or have a honeycomb appearance. Moreover, a SCA would be suspected if there is a central scar, which is found in less than 30% of SCAs (**Figure 1.10**).
- A mucinous cystic neoplasm (MCN) fits nicely: middle-aged woman, at the tail of the pancreas, no ductal connection, usually unilocular or thinly septated. These do have malignant potential, but not all are dangerous. However, if the cyst was

larger, then EUS and/or surgical consultation after discussion at a multidisciplinary conference would be indicated (**Figure 1.11**).

- A side-branch (aka branch-duct) IPMN is possible here. Those side branches communicate with the main pancreatic duct, and can occur anywhere in the pancreas, including the tail (**Figure 1.12**). These can also be multifocal and less commonly unilocular compared with MCN.
- The cyst might also be a pseudocyst, but without a history of pancreatitis or trauma, that's unlikely.

Figure 1.10. *Serous cystadenoma. (A) CT scan showing 5-cm SCA with numerous microcysts and central calcification in the pancreatic tail. (B) Gross pathology of SCA showing the classic microcystic honeycomb appearance with a central stellate scar.*[36]

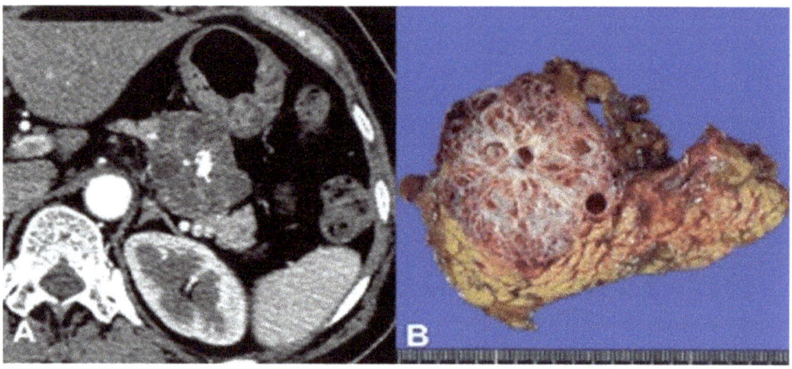

Figure 1.11. *Mucinous cystic neoplasm. (A) CT scan showing 4.5-cm MCN in the pancreatic tail. (B) A multilocular cyst with septa noted. (C) Gross pathology of MCN with macrocysts separated by fibrous septa.*[36]

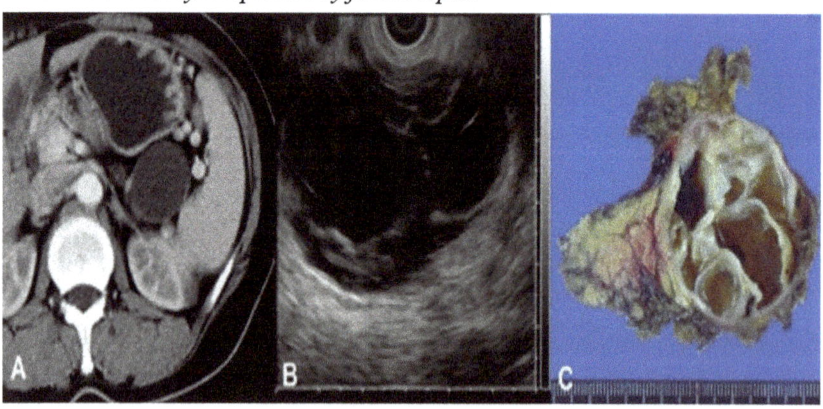

Figure 1.12. *Side-branch IPMN. T2-weighted MRI of 2.1-cm side-branch IPMN (arrow) noted in the pancreatic tail without alarm features.*[37]

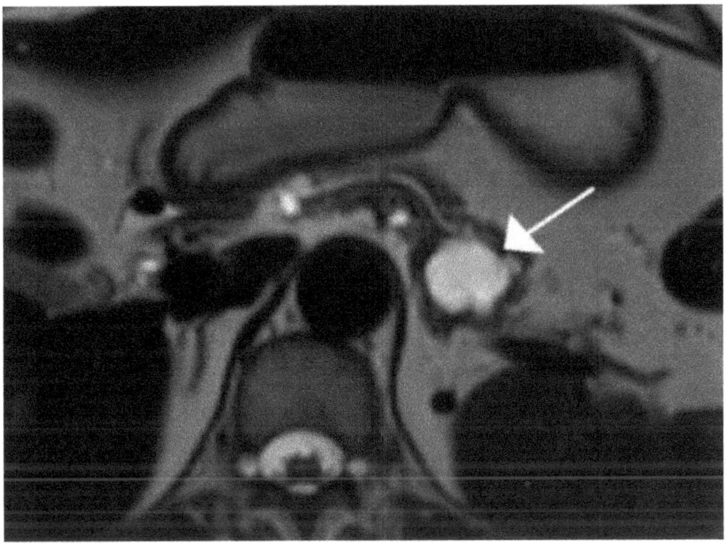

Bottom line: We're likely dealing with an MCN, or less likely a side-branch IPMN or SCA. But classification isn't our priority yet—risk stratification is. See **Table 1.7** for a breakdown of all the different pancreatic cysts. This table is solid gold!

Step 2: Is it worrisome?

Pancreatic cysts can be divided into 3 risk tiers: high-risk stigmata, which generally trigger surgery; worrisome features, which prompt EUS ± FNA; and low-risk features, which can usually be followed with imaging alone. The key is to match the patient's cyst to the corresponding column in **Table 1.8** and act accordingly.

Table 1.7. *Key Characteristics of Four Pancreatic Cysts.*

Cyst type	Gender	Age	Imaging Description	Cytology/Markers	Malignant Potential
Mucinous cystic neoplam	More in females	Middle-aged	98% body or tail; thick mucin	CEA > 192; low amylase	Moderate
IPMN (intraductal papillary mucinous neoplasm)	No gender bias	Middle-aged to older	"Fishmouth," "cluster of grapes"	CEA > 192; high amylase	Variable
Serous cystadenoma	More in females	Older	Microcystic or honeycomb; central scar	Low CEA (<0.5); +glycogen (cuboidal cells)	Way low
Solid pseudopapillary neoplasm	Females (95%)	Young (< 40 yrs)	Mixed solid/cystic; in body/tail	Low CEA; branching "finger-like" projections	Moderate

Table 1.8. *Pancreatic Cyst Risk Features.*

High-Risk Features	Worrisome Features	Low-Risk Features
* Enhancing solid component * Main PD ≥10 mm * Obstructive jaundice + head cyst	* Cyst ≥3 cm * Mural nodule * Thickened/enhancing wall * Main PD 5-9 mm * Abrupt Main PD caliber change * Lymphadenopathy * Rapid growth (>5 mm/year) * Elevated CA 19-9 * Unexplained pancreatitis	* Cyst <3 cm * No nodules * Thin-walled, simple cyst * Normal duct size * No ductal changes * No lymph nodes * Stable size * Normal CA 19-9 * No history of pancreatitis

This patient, in general, has low-risk features. Her cyst is under 3 cm with no nodules and no thickening. She has a normal pancreatic duct and no symptoms and no elevated tumor markers. However, you also don't know whether this is a mucinous or non-mucinous cyst. So, it is certainly reasonable in this particular case to proceed with an EUS now to figure out whether you are dealing with a mucinous cyst or not. If it is mucinous, then you need to track it. However, you don't need to follow up a non-mucinous cyst (such as an SCA).

In general, a cyst <3 cm is less worrisome, but it all depends. Know Table 1.7!

Step 3: How to follow it

This is where good medicine becomes good stewardship. Surveillance isn't about chasing every cyst—it's about watching for evolution. The ACG guideline recommends that for cysts 2–3 cm with no worrisome features, follow-up imaging should be done in 1 year, then every 2 years thereafter if the cyst remains stable.

Small cyst with no worrisome features? Image in 1 year, then every 2 years if stable.

MRI or MRCP is the preferred imaging modality—not CT—

because it gives better definition of the cyst wall, septations, and ductal anatomy, without radiation exposure. And unlike EUS, it doesn't require sedation or a procedure room.

The big question patients often ask is: *How long do I have to keep getting these scans?* The current ACG guideline says that it is reasonable to stop surveillance for those older than 75 years old and certainly if the patient is no longer a surgical candidate. Interestingly, the American Gastroenterological Association guideline slightly differs and suggests that you can quit surveillance if the cyst remains stable over 5 years.[38] For a healthy 63-year-old, you might extend that window a bit longer.

Let her know that any new symptoms—pain, jaundice, pancreatitis, weight loss—would reset the clock. That's not surveillance failure—it's your cue to reevaluate and possibly escalate.

Bringing It Together

This is a low-risk, asymptomatic, incidental cyst in a woman with no red flags and a clean scan. It's most likely an MCN, which requires follow-up (MRI in 1 year, then every 2 years if stable). However, an EUS can be done now to determine the need for long-term surveillance. That is, if the cyst turns out to be non-mucinous, such as an SCA, then there is no need to surveil any further.

Pancreas Quiz

1. A 47-year-old woman presents with sudden-onset severe epigastric pain radiating to the back. Her serum lipase is 1,250 U/L (normal < 80). CT abdomen performed in the ED shows mild stranding around the pancreas but no fluid collection or necrosis. She is afebrile, hemodynamically stable, and has normal renal function. Which of the following statements best reflects guideline-based management at this stage?

   a. A contrast-enhanced CT is necessary to confirm the diagnosis before initiating treatment
   b. An amylase level should also be obtained to meet diagnostic criteria
   c. Imaging findings of necrosis are essential to distinguish acute from chronic pancreatitis
   d. No further imaging is needed now, as clinical and laboratory criteria are sufficient to make the diagnosis
   e. Lipase levels must exceed 5× ULN to meet diagnostic threshold

2. A 55-year-old woman presents with epigastric abdominal pain radiating to the back. She is nauseated but hemodynamically stable. Her serum amylase is 210 U/L (normal <140), and lipase was not ordered. CT imaging has not yet been performed. What is the most appropriate next step?

   a. Order a lipase level to clarify the diagnosis
   b. Proceed with supportive care for acute pancreatitis
   c. Order contrast-enhanced CT to assess for inflammation
   d. Repeat amylase in 6 hours
   e. Exclude pancreatitis based on borderline enzyme levels

3. A 60-year-old man presents with upper abdominal pain and nausea. Labs show a lipase of 165 U/L (normal <80) and an amylase of 140 U/L. The pain is poorly localized and non-radiating. He has mild leukocytosis but no fever. You are uncertain whether the pain is pancreatic in origin. What is the most appropriate next step?

   a. Begin IV fluids and observe—no further testing needed
   b. Diagnose acute pancreatitis and admit for supportive care
   c. Order contrast-enhanced CT to evaluate for acute pancreatitis
   d. Order stool elastase to assess for chronic pancreatitis
   e. Repeat lipase and amylase in 24 hours

4. A 50-year-old man is admitted with acute pancreatitis. He has no history of alcohol use, no gallstones on ultrasound, and no prior episodes. Lipid panel and calcium are normal. ALT is 18 U/L. He is hemodynamically stable, tolerating oral intake by day 2 According to ACG guidelines, what is the next best step in evaluating the cause of his pancreatitis?

   a. No further testing is needed unless recurrence occurs
   b. Order EUS or MRCP to evaluate for occult biliary disease
   c. Schedule ERCP to assess for choledocholithiasis
   d. Begin empiric steroids for presumed autoimmune pancreatitis
   e. Perform CT-guided FNA to evaluate for pancreatic infection

5. A 45-year-old woman is admitted with her first episode of acute pancreatitis. She denies alcohol use and takes no regular medications. Her triglycerides and calcium are normal. Lipase is 920 U/L. A CT abdomen shows pancreatic edema, but no stones or ductal dilation. ALT is 65 U/L. She is recovering well with supportive care. What is the most appropriate next step to evaluate etiology?

   a. No further workup is needed—idiopathic pancreatitis is likely
   b. Order MRCP to evaluate for ductal strictures
   c. Schedule genetic testing
   d. Obtain right upper quadrant ultrasound
   e. Start antibiotics for presumed biliary infection

6. A 57-year-old woman is admitted with acute pancreatitis. She does not drink alcohol. Labs reveal lipase >3× ULN, ALT 42 U/L, triglycerides 260 mg/dL, and corrected calcium 9.2 mg/dL. Right upper quadrant ultrasound shows no gallstones and a normal common bile duct. Her CT scan shows pancreatic edema but no masses or collections. This is her first episode. The team concludes the case is idiopathic and plans discharge without further testing. According to the ACG guidelines, which of the following best reflects the optimal next step?

   a. Consider as idiopathic only if MRCP or EUS is unrevealing after recovery
   b. Order ERCP to evaluate for occult biliary pathology
   c. Repeat ultrasound in 3 months before labeling as idiopathic
   d. Check serum IgG4 and consider steroids for autoimmune pancreatitis
   e. Proceed with genetic testing due to lack of identifiable etiology

7. A 36-year-old man is admitted with acute pancreatitis. He has no prior medical history. He is afebrile, mildly tachycardic, and his initial hematocrit is 44%. BUN is 17 mg/dL. He receives a 1-liter bolus of lactated Ringer's followed by 150 mL/hour. Six hours later, his hematocrit is 46% and BUN is 23 mg/dL. He is not short of breath and has good urine output. According to the ACG guidelines, what is the most appropriate next step in his management?

   a. Continue current fluid rate—he is improving
   b. Repeat CT scan to assess for early necrosis
   c. Increase fluid rate to 2–3 mL/kg/hour and monitor closely
   d. Reduce fluid rate to avoid overload
   e. Switch to normal saline for broader electrolyte coverage

8. A 42-year-old woman is admitted with moderate acute pancreatitis. She is started on intravenous normal saline at 200 mL/hour. You are consulted twelve hours into her hospitalization and suggest switching to lactated Ringer's. Which of the following best explains the rationale for preferring lactated Ringer's in this setting?

   a. It improves pancreatic enzyme clearance
   b. It is less likely to cause hyperkalemia
   c. It reduces the need for early antibiotic therapy
   d. It is associated with lower systemic inflammation in early pancreatitis
   e. It decreases splanchnic blood flow less than normal saline

9. A 50-year-old man is admitted with acute pancreatitis. He is started on lactated Ringer's at 150 mL/hour. His hematocrit is 43% on admission and 41% at 12 hours. His BUN is stable at 19 mg/dL. He is breathing comfortably, has adequate urine output, and his vitals are stable. According to the ACG guidelines, what is the most appropriate next step?

   a. Bolus an additional 2 liters of fluid to accelerate hemodilution
   b. Continue current fluid rate and monitor trends
   c. Reduce fluid rate to avoid fluid overload
   d. Switch to normal saline for more sodium support
   e. Order early CT to rule out necrosis

10. A 58-year-old man with severe acute pancreatitis undergoes CT imaging on hospital day 4, which reveals a large area of non-enhancing pancreatic parenchyma and a small peripancreatic fluid collection. He is febrile to 100.9°F but hemodynamically stable, with improving leukocytosis and good pain control. There is no gas in the collection. According to the ACG guidelines, what is the most appropriate next step?

    a. Start broad-spectrum antibiotics to prevent infection
    b. Refer to surgery for early necrosectomy
    c. Begin enteral nutrition and continue supportive care
    d. Order CT-guided FNA to rule out infected necrosis
    e. Switch to total parenteral nutrition to rest the pancreas

11. A male patient with acute pancreatitis is found on day 5 to have non-enhancing pancreatic necrosis on CT. He is afebrile, hemodynamically stable, and recovering with supportive care. The primary team wants to begin empiric antibiotics. According to ACG guidelines, which of the following best describes the role of antibiotics in this setting?

    a. Antibiotics reduce the risk of infected necrosis and should be started prophylactically
    b. Antibiotics should be given only if there is gas in the collection or clinical signs of infection
    c. Carbapenems should be started now, as necrosis has been confirmed radiographically
    d. Antibiotics are recommended for all patients with necrosis >30% of the gland
    e. Empiric antibiotics are appropriate while awaiting repeat imaging

12. A 61-year-old man with severe acute pancreatitis is found to have necrosis involving >50% of the pancreas. On day 6, he is febrile and has mild leukocytosis but is stable on room air, tolerating some oral intake, and has no signs of organ failure. CT shows a non-enhancing area of necrosis without gas or defined fluid collection. According to the ACG guidelines, what is the most appropriate management approach?

    a. Begin drainage now to prevent later infected necrosis
    b. Schedule endoscopic debridement within 1 week
    c. Repeat CT-guided FNA to confirm sterile necrosis
    d. Continue supportive care without intervention at this stage
    e. Refer for urgent surgical necrosectomy

13. A 58-year-old man with necrotizing pancreatitis develops fever and leukocytosis on hospital day 19. A repeat CT shows a large walled-off necrotic collection with internal gas bubbles. He is hemodynamically stable on room air. Which of the following is the next best step in management?

    a. Start broad-spectrum antibiotics and monitor without immediate drainage
    b. Schedule surgical necrosectomy within 24 hours
    c. Repeat FNA to confirm infection before starting antibiotics
    d. Begin empiric antifungal therapy
    e. Delay intervention for at least 4 weeks and avoid all antibiotics unless unstable

14. A patient with infected pancreatic necrosis is started on meropenem after a CT shows gas within a walled-off collection. After 72 hours of antibiotics, he remains febrile and is now requiring vasopressors. What is the most appropriate next step?

    a. Continue antibiotics for 7 more days before considering drainage
    b. Refer for surgical necrosectomy as the first intervention
    c. Begin step-up therapy with percutaneous drainage
    d. Switch to oral antibiotics and monitor
    e. Start corticosteroids to reduce inflammation before intervention

15. A 62-year-old man with infected necrotizing pancreatitis undergoes percutaneous drainage on day 30 of illness but remains septic. The collection is well-formed and walled-off. The team is planning endoscopic necrosectomy the next day. What is the main rationale for delaying invasive debridement until this stage?

    a. It allows pancreatic enzyme levels to normalize before intervention
    b. It improves accuracy of culture results from the collection
    c. It reduces bleeding risk by allowing pseudocyst encapsulation
    d. It allows necrosis to liquefy and wall off, improving procedural safety and success
    e. It prevents antibiotic resistance from prolonged empiric therapy

16. A 55-year-old woman presents with gallstone pancreatitis. She is afebrile, mildly tachycardic, and jaundiced. Labs reveal WBC 13.2, total bilirubin 3.5 mg/dL, and ALT 210 U/L. CT abdomen shows peripancreatic stranding, and ultrasound reveals gallstones but no

ductal dilation. She is hemodynamically stable and not hypoxic. According to the ACG guidelines, what is the most appropriate next step regarding ERCP?

a. Proceed with urgent ERCP within 24 hours
b. Defer ERCP and obtain EUS or MRCP to assess for ductal stones
c. ERCP is not indicated—repeat imaging in 1 week
d. Schedule cholecystectomy before imaging the duct
e. Start empiric antibiotics and proceed to ERCP once afebrile

17. A patient with confirmed choledocholithiasis is scheduled for ERCP. She has no history of kidney disease or NSAID allergy. According to ACG guidelines, which of the following strategies should be used to reduce the risk of post-ERCP pancreatitis?

a. IV corticosteroids 30 minutes before the procedure
b. Antibiotics and fasting for 24 hours prior to ERCP
c. Rectal indomethacin 100 mg and aggressive IV hydration with lactated Ringer's
d. Oral acetaminophen and placement of a pancreatic duct stent
e. Intramuscular meperidine and intra-rectal ice packs

18. A 60-year-old man presents with right upper quadrant pain, fever, and jaundice—fulfilling Charcot's triad. He also appears confused and is hypotensive on arrival. Which of the following two additional findings completes Reynold's pentad, indicating severe suppurative cholangitis?

a. Leukocytosis and elevated alkaline phosphatase
b. Vomiting and dehydration
c. Hypoxia and elevated lipase
d. Weight loss and fatigue
e. Mental status changes and hypotension

19. A 40-year-old man presents with his third episode of acute pancreatitis. Prior evaluations have shown normal ultrasound, triglycerides, calcium, and no history of alcohol or medications. CT scan showed no stones or mass. He is otherwise healthy and has no family history of pancreatitis. What is the best next step in evaluation?

a. Repeat CT to reassess for subtle inflammation
b. Label the case idiopathic and begin chronic pain management
c. Obtain EUS or MRCP
d. Refer for diagnostic ERCP
e. Begin empirical pancreatic enzyme therapy

20. A 34-year-old woman with no alcohol use or gallstones has had 2 hospitalizations for acute pancreatitis. Ultrasound, triglycerides, calcium, and MRCP have all been unremarkable. She has no personal history of cystic fibrosis but recalls that her brother had recurrent "stomach problems" in his 20s. Fecal elastase is normal. Which of the following is the best next step in her workup?

    a. Pancreatic biopsy for autoimmune pancreatitis
    b. Trial of pancreatic enzyme therapy
    c. Cholecystectomy to reduce recurrence
    d. Empiric steroid therapy
    e. Genetic testing for *PRSS1, SPINK1, CFTR*, and *CTRC* mutations

21. A 52-year-old man with no identifiable etiology has been hospitalized twice in the past year for acute pancreatitis. Ultrasound, EUS, labs, and MRCP have all failed to reveal gallstones, sludge, elevated triglycerides, or ductal abnormalities. He is otherwise healthy and has no family history of pancreatic disease. According to the ACG guidelines, which of the following is an appropriate management option?

    a. Empiric cholecystectomy may be considered to reduce recurrence
    b. Repeat CT every 6 months to monitor for evolving pathology
    c. Begin pancreatic enzyme therapy and schedule ERCP
    d. Label as idiopathic and monitor for chronic pancreatitis
    e. Avoid surgery unless future episodes involve necrosis

22. A 45-year-old man has had recurrent postprandial epigastric pain for years. He has no alcohol use, normal labs, and normal CT. Fecal elastase is borderline at 190 μg/g. EGD is unremarkable. You suspect early chronic pancreatitis. According to the ACG guidelines, what is the best next diagnostic step?
    a. Diagnose functional dyspepsia and initiate neuromodulators
    b. Perform endoscopic ultrasound to assess for subtle parenchymal and ductal changes
    c. Begin pancreatic enzyme therapy for pain management
    d. Label the case idiopathic and observe for exocrine insufficiency
    e. Proceed to genetic testing to evaluate for hereditary CP

23. Which of the following best reflects the current ACG guideline definition of chronic pancreatitis?

    a. Chronic pancreatitis is diagnosed by the presence of pancreatic calcifications or ductal abnormalities on imaging
    b. Chronic pancreatitis is defined as recurrent pancreatitis with evidence of exocrine insufficiency
    c. Chronic pancreatitis is confirmed by a fecal elastase < 200 μg/g with symptoms of steatorrhea
    d. Chronic pancreatitis is a progressive fibro-inflammatory syndrome characterized by loss of function and structural damage
    e. Chronic pancreatitis can only be diagnosed histologically

24. A 45-year-old man with suspected early chronic pancreatitis on EUS has a fecal elastase level of 205 μg/g. He has experienced weight loss and postprandial abdominal discomfort, but no steatorrhea. Which of the following statements is the most accurate regarding fecal elastase testing?

    a. A result >200 μg/g definitively excludes exocrine pancreatic insufficiency
    b. Fecal elastase testing is the gold standard for diagnosing chronic pancreatitis
    c. Borderline results like this warrant consideration of a trial of pancreatic enzyme therapy
    d. Elastase levels are more useful than EUS for diagnosing early chronic pancreatitis
    e. Fecal elastase levels are falsely low in patients with pancreatic divisum

25. A 47-year-old man with recurrent postprandial epigastric pain undergoes EUS for suspected chronic pancreatitis. The exam reveals 3 parenchymal features (lobularity, echogenic foci, and strands) and 1 ductal feature (main duct irregularity). Fecal elastase is 210 μg/g. CT and MRI were previously normal. According to the ACG guidelines, what is the most appropriate next step?

    a. Diagnose chronic pancreatitis and initiate long-term enzyme therapy
    b. Order s-MRCP to further evaluate ductal anatomy and function
    c. Label the case as functional dyspepsia and discontinue GI workup
    d. Proceed to pancreatic biopsy for confirmation
    e. Begin corticosteroids for presumed autoimmune pancreatitis

26. A 52-year-old woman with bloating and intermittent abdominal discomfort undergoes EUS. The study shows two minor parenchymal features—mild lobularity and a few echogenic strands. Fecal elastase is normal, and she has no history of pancreatitis, weight loss, or malabsorption. CT and MRI were both normal. According to the ACG guidelines, how should this EUS result be interpreted?

    a. Findings are diagnostic for chronic pancreatitis
    b. Minor EUS features confirm early exocrine dysfunction
    c. These findings may occur in normal individuals and should not prompt diagnosis of CP
    d. A Rosemont score is needed to assess disease stage
    e. Corticosteroids should be started empirically for subclinical autoimmune pancreatitis

27. A 46-year-old man with recurrent epigastric pain and weight loss undergoes EUS, which shows two parenchymal features and one ductal feature suggestive but not definitive for chronic pancreatitis. CT is normal. Fecal elastase is 225 μg/g. The gastroenterology team is unsure how to proceed. According to the ACG guidelines, what is the most appropriate next step?

    a. Start enzyme therapy and monitor for symptom improvement
    b. Label the case as minimal change chronic pancreatitis and initiate long-term follow-up
    c. Obtain secretin-enhanced MRCP to assess ductal function and structure
    d. Proceed to pancreatic biopsy to confirm fibrosis
    e. Repeat EUS in 6 months to assess for progression

28. A 49-year-old woman is diagnosed with early chronic pancreatitis based on symptoms, borderline fecal elastase, and imaging findings on s-MRCP. She does not drink alcohol or smoke, and there is no history of gallstones or pancreatitis. Which of the following frameworks do the ACG guidelines recommend using to guide etiologic evaluation?

    a. RANSON
    b. ROSEWOOD
    c. M-ANNHEIM
    d. TIGAR-O
    e. Atlanta 1996

29. A 45-year-old man with early chronic pancreatitis suggested on imaging has a fecal elastase of 185 μg/g. He reports a 12-pound weight loss over the past 6 months but denies diarrhea or steatorrhea. He is otherwise stable. According to ACG guidelines, what is the most appropriate next step?

    a. Begin pancreatic enzyme therapy due to evidence of early exocrine insufficiency
    b. Delay therapy until fecal elastase falls below 100 μg/g
    c. Initiate corticosteroids for presumed autoimmune pancreatitis
    d. Enzyme therapy is not helpful unless pain is the dominant symptom
    e. Order ERCP to confirm diagnosis before starting treatment

30. A 52-year-old woman has recently been diagnosed with chronic pancreatitis. She has mild weight loss, borderline fecal elastase, and a stable HbA1c. She is started on pancreatic enzyme therapy and doing well clinically. According to ACG guidelines, which of the following is part of appropriate long-term monitoring?

    a. Repeat CT imaging every 12 months to monitor for progression
    b. Annual serum amylase and lipase to assess disease activity
    c. ERCP to evaluate for asymptomatic ductal strictures
    d. Routine stool fat testing to assess for malabsorption
    e. Bone mineral density (DEXA) screening every 2–3 years

31. A 58-year-old man with chronic pancreatitis has persistent postprandial epigastric pain despite abstaining from alcohol and smoking. He is on high-dose pancreatic enzymes and acid suppression. CT reveals a dilated pancreatic duct measuring 7 mm with small stones. According to the ACG guidelines, what is the best next step in managing his pain?

    a. Refer for endoscopic ductal decompression
    b. Increase enzyme dose to further reduce pancreatic stimulation
    c. Add antioxidant therapy and continue conservative management
    d. Proceed directly to surgical drainage
    e. Begin opioid therapy for long-term symptom control

32. A patient with chronic pancreatitis has ongoing pain and is on a high-dose pancreatic enzyme regimen. His weight is stable, vitamin levels are normal, and there are no signs of steatorrhea or malabsorption. He asks whether increasing the enzyme dose might help with pain control. According to the ACG guidelines, what is the most appropriate response?

    a. Increase enzyme dose and add a proton pump inhibitor
    b. Enzymes reduce pancreatic stimulation and are first-line for pain
    c. Continue current dose—enzymes are not indicated for pain in the absence of EPI
    d. Discontinue enzymes—long-term use increases ductal pressure
    e. Add corticosteroids to reduce pancreatic inflammation

33. A 54-year-old woman with chronic pancreatitis and persistent epigastric pain has failed lifestyle modification, enzyme therapy, and a trial of antioxidants. Imaging shows a dilated pancreatic duct with intraductal calcifications. She is now requiring escalating doses of opioids and asks about surgical options. According to the ACG guidelines, what is the best next step in management?

    a. Refer for surgical drainage since medical therapy has failed
    b. Consider endoscopic decompression before surgical referral
    c. Begin tricyclic antidepressants for functional overlay
    d. Continue opioid therapy and schedule CT in 6 months
    e. Refer for total pancreatectomy with islet autotransplantation (TPIAT)

34. A 66-year-old man is admitted with painless jaundice. CT shows a diffusely enlarged pancreas without a discrete mass. Labs show elevated total IgG, a positive ANA, and normal IgG4. He reports recent weight loss and dry mouth. ALT and bilirubin are elevated. There is no history of pancreatitis or alcohol use. What is the most appropriate next step?

    a. Refer for Whipple procedure due to suspicion for pancreatic cancer
    b. Label as chronic pancreatitis and begin enzyme therapy
    c. Repeat CT in 1 month to assess for progression
    d. Order EUS-guided FNA to confirm malignancy
    e. Begin diagnostic steroid trial and monitor for response

35. A 63-year-old woman is found to have a 3.2-cm unilocular pancreatic cyst in the tail on CT performed for unrelated abdominal pain. She is asymptomatic, with no family history of pancreatic cancer. The cyst has no mural nodule, normal duct, and is described as thin-walled. What is the best next step?

    a. Order EUS with FNA to assess for mucinous content
    b. Refer for surgical resection due to risk of malignancy
    c. Begin annual CT surveillance with contrast
    d. Repeat imaging in 1 year, then every 2 years if stable
    e. Schedule ERCP to evaluate ductal anatomy

36. A 55-year-old man is found to have a 2.8-cm pancreatic cyst in the head of the pancreas during workup for vague abdominal discomfort. He has a remote history of gallstone pancreatitis. MRI shows a multiloculated cyst with communication to the pancreatic duct and no mural nodules. Fluid analysis shows CEA 300 ng/mL and high amylase. Cytology is negative. Which of the following is the most likely diagnosis?

    a. Serous cystadenoma
    b. Pseudocyst
    c. Mucinous cystic neoplasm
    d. Intraductal papillary mucinous neoplasm (IPMN)
    e. Solid pseudopapillary neoplasm

Answers to Pancreas Guidelines Quiz

1.	D	19.	C
2.	A	20.	E
3.	C	21.	A
4.	B	22.	B
5.	D	23.	D
6.	A	24.	C
7.	C	25.	B
8.	D	26.	C
9.	B	27.	C
10.	C	28.	D
11.	B	29.	A
12.	D	30.	E
13.	A	31.	A
14.	C	32.	C
15.	D	33.	B
16.	B	34.	E
17.	C	35.	A
18.	E	36.	D

Chapter Two

BILE AND BRIMSTONE

A Guide to Biliary Mayhem

The liver's drainage system looks simple on the diagram—one green line flowing neatly into another—but in real life, it can behave like a garden hose with kinks, rust, and a mind of its own. When that happens, even the calmest GI doc can start Googling airfare to an island getaway.

In this chapter, we'll wrestle with 2 heavyweight ACG guidelines:

1. **Benign and Malignant Biliary Strictures** – When to brush, when to biopsy, when to stent, when to call interventional radiology, and when to call your momma before your patient's bilirubin starts plotting a hostile takeover.
2. **Primary Sclerosing Cholangitis (PSC)** – The maddening cousin of IBD that can turn ducts into crepe paper and make seasoned hepatologists reach for the antacids.

Expect cameo appearances by dominant strictures, IgG4 impostors, gallbladder polyps that overstay their welcome, and the eternal "stent or not" debate. We'll decode fluorescence in situ hybridization (FISH) polysomy without dredging up your freshman genetics nightmares, show why high-dose ursodeoxycholic acid (UDCA) went from hero to outlaw, and remind you (often) that an 8-mm gallbladder polyp in PSC is about as soothing as a smoke alarm at 3 AM.

So, grab your scope, your best duct-taming playlist, and a healthy respect for bile gone bad. Time to dive into biliary mayhem.

Case 2.1: Is It Cancer?

A 67-year-old man presents to clinic with progressive painless jaundice over the past 3 weeks. He also notes dark urine, mild pruritus, and an unintended 15-pound weight loss over 2 months. He has not experienced fever or abdominal pain. Laboratory tests reveal a total bilirubin of 6.3 mg/dL, elevated alkaline phosphatase, and mildly elevated transaminases. CA 19-9 is 110 U/mL.

Abdominal ultrasound reveals dilated intrahepatic bile ducts and a distended gallbladder. A contrast-enhanced CT scan shows a 1.8 cm area of ill-defined soft tissue at the distal common bile duct near the head of the pancreas, concerning for malignancy.

You are now consulted to assist with diagnosis and management.

Know your guidelines!

1. What is the preferred initial diagnostic approach for this suspected malignant extrahepatic biliary stricture?
2. Should ERCP or EUS come first?
3. What is the role of tissue acquisition — and what techniques are most appropriate?
4. Should biliary drainage be performed now or deferred?
5. If this is ultimately found to be resectable pancreatic cancer, what does the guideline say about stenting?

Case 2.1: What do the guidelines say?

Source: ACG 2023 Management of Biliary Strictures Guideline[39]

This is the kind of case that should light up your internal alarm system. An older patient with painless jaundice, dark urine, pruritus, and weight loss is a walking case study in obstructive jaundice from a malignant biliary stricture. And indeed, the CT suggests a soft tissue lesion near the pancreatic head — pushing pancreatic cancer high on the list. But let's not be too quick to close the book on the differential.

The causes of biliary strictures are broader than we often give them credit for. Sure, malignancy tops the list — pancreatic cancer and cholangiocarcinoma are the leading culprits — depending on location. But benign etiologies are far from rare, and autoimmune, infectious, or post-surgical causes can muddy the waters. Don't forget to keep your view wide before you narrow in, especially if tissue sampling later proves inconclusive.

"Painless jaundice" should make you think about cancer. But remember, the differential diagnosis includes benign etiologies too

The CA 19-9 of 110 U/mL may seem to reinforce the malignancy theory, but it's a slippery marker. CA 19-9 lacks specificity and can be elevated in a variety of benign and malignant conditions — some of which have nothing to do with cancer. Also important: about 5%–10% of patients don't secrete CA 19-9 at all, so a normal value doesn't rule out cancer either. **Table 2.1** shows

CA 19-9 lacks specificity for cancer and can be elevated with many conditions

Table 2.1 *Common Causes of Elevated CA 19-9 (i.e., it's not just cancer).*

Category	Examples
Malignancy	Pancreatic adenocarcinoma, cholangiocarcinoma, gastric cancer, hepatocellular carcinoma, ovarian cancer
Benign hepatobiliary disease	Obstructive jaundice, cholestasis, cirrhosis, primary sclerosing cholangitis
Pancreatic disorders	Acute or chronic pancreatitis
Autoimmune disease	IgG4-related sclerosing cholangitis
Infection	Hepatitis, cholangitis, TB (rare)
Other	Cystic fibrosis, diabetes (rare reports)

the more common causes of elevated CA 19-9 — a reminder that interpreting this test in isolation is a rookie mistake.

EUS First Because It Outperforms ERCP for Diagnosis

Worried about an obstructive mass? EUS is the preferred first test

Now comes the critical decision: how do we confirm the diagnosis and obtain tissue? While ERCP is tempting for its dual diagnostic and therapeutic potential, the ACG guidelines make this call easy: EUS is preferred as the initial diagnostic modality when a mass is suspected or seen on imaging.

Why? Because it performs better. EUS with FNA or fine needle biopsy (FNB) achieves higher sensitivity for malignancy—up to 95%—when a mass is clearly visualized. ERCP, by contrast, suffers from poor sensitivity despite high specificity.[40] A positive brushing can clinch the diagnosis, sure, but a negative one doesn't rule it out. That's a dangerous blind spot when you're trying to move quickly toward definitive treatment.

Equally important is the order of operations. If you're planning both EUS and ERCP, they should ideally be done in a single session—but EUS should come first. ERCP introduces contrast and mechanical trauma to the ducts, which can cause edema, inflammation, or even post-ERCP pancreatitis. These changes can obscure the EUS field and reduce the quality or safety of FNA/FNB. So, unless logistics absolutely preclude it, the sequence should ideally be: EUS first, ERCP second, preferably in the same sitting if possible.

In this case, with a distal biliary lesion and clear mass effect on imaging, EUS-FNA/FNB gives the best chance at an early, definitive diagnosis — and a cleaner roadmap to surgical decision-making.

Don't Rush to Drain — Unless There's a Real Need

Once the diagnosis is confirmed — or even if you're still in workup mode — the next question is whether to stent. It's a tempting reflex: jaundiced patient, high bilirubin, why not decompress? But here's where a little restraint can save your patient from harm. The guidelines don't want us rushing to a stent straight off the bat.

Routine pre-operative biliary drainage is not recommended for patients with clearly resectable disease unless there is a specific clinical need. And that's not just a theoretical stance — it's grounded in trial data. Pre-op stenting has been associated with increased infectious complications, delayed time to surgery, and technical issues during resection.[40] It can contaminate an otherwise clean field and lead to stent occlusion or cholangitis, all before a scalpel ever touches the skin.

Routine preop biliary drainage is not recommended for patients with resectable pancreatic cancer

So, when should you stent? Only when necessary. If the patient is cholangitic, then obviously it's warranted to mitigate sepsis and save life. If there is intractable pruritus, or the bilirubin is high enough (e.g. > 14 mg/dL), then you may need to decompress. Also, if the patient cannot undergo surgery , then you may also need to decompress. Also, if the patient cannot undergo surgery promptly — say, due to transfer delays, cardiac clearance, or the need for neoadjuvant therapy — then biliary drainage becomes more reasonable.

Indications for stenting:

* Cholangitis
* Bad pruritis
* Bilirubin > 14
* Barriers to timely surgery

And when you do decide to stent, choose wisely. There are differences. For example, fully-covered self-expanding metal stents (fcSEMS) typically offer longer patency, fewer occlusions, and easier removability than uncovered SEMS. SEMS also clog less frequently than plastic stents. However, plastic stents still have a role in short-term decompression or when there's concern about covering the cystic duct or in settings of altered anatomy.

If you're going to stent a malignant stricture, SEMS are favored over plastic stents

Bringing It Together

In the evaluation of a suspected malignant extrahepatic biliary stricture, particularly with an identifiable mass, EUS with FNA/FNB should be your first step. It's safer, more accurate, and less invasive than ERCP, and should precede it when both are being done. Ideally, they occur in a single session — but always in the right order.

Avoid reflexive stenting. Unless the patient is systemically ill, symptomatic, or facing surgical delays, hold off. And when you do place a stent, pick the right tool. SEMS are usually favored over plastic in most of these scenarios, unless a specific anatomic or clinical factor pushes you otherwise.

Case 2.2: Stricture Without a Verdict

A 72-year-old woman presents with progressive jaundice, fatigue, and a 10-pound weight loss over the past 2 months. Her medical history is notable for hypertension, hypothyroidism, and remote cholecystectomy. She has no history of pancreatitis, autoimmune disease, or IBD.

Labs reveal a total bilirubin of 7.2 mg/dL, with elevated alkaline phosphatase and mild transaminemia.* CA 19-9 is 65 U/mL.

Abdominal ultrasound shows intrahepatic biliary dilation. MRCP confirms a high-grade stricture in the mid-common bile duct without a clear mass. She undergoes ERCP (**Figure 2.1**) with brush cytology and forceps biopsies. Both return as non-diagnostic — atypical cells, suspicious but not definitive.

Figure 2.1. *ERCP with high-grade stricture in common bile duct.*

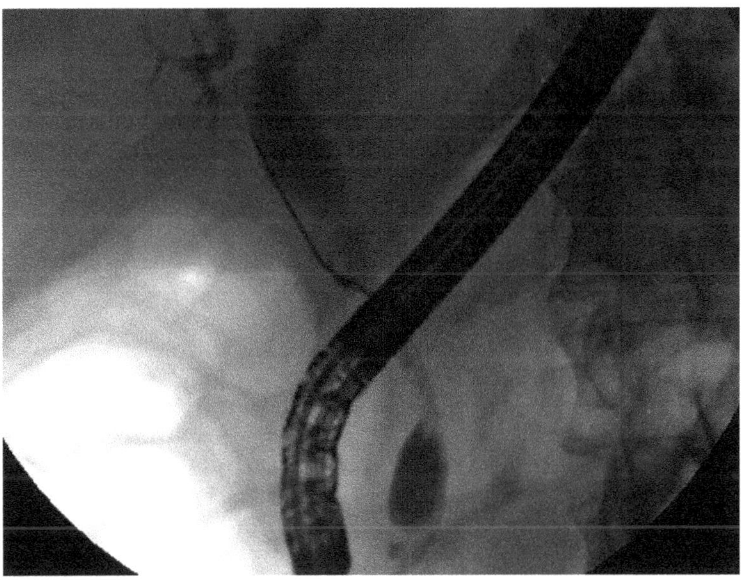

* That's right, we said "transaminemia," not "transaminitis," which literally means "inflammation of the transaminases." That term doesn't make sense, despite most everyone using it in clinical practice.

The clinical team is unsure whether to escalate to cholangioscopy, refer for EUS, repeat ERCP, get a FISH analysis, discuss surgical exploration, or just go home for the day and watch ESPN.

Know your guidelines!

1. What should be the next step after nondiagnostic ERCP sampling in an indeterminate biliary stricture?
2. When should you add cholangioscopy or FISH analysis?
3. What's the role of EUS when there's no visible mass on imaging?
4. At what point do we throw in the towel and call for tumor board or surgery?

Case 2.2: What do the guidelines say?
Source: ACG 2023 Management of Biliary Strictures Guidelines[39]

This is a patient with obstructive jaundice, intrahepatic dilation, and a common bile duct stricture—but no discrete mass and inconclusive tissue sampling. It's what the guideline terms an "indeterminate biliary stricture"—defined as a stricture that persists despite prior negative or nondiagnostic workup, including cross-sectional imaging and initial endoscopic tissue acquisition.

When you find yourself staring at atypical brushings or benign-looking forceps biopsy results—and you're still worried—you've entered this gray zone. And here's the key: a negative result doesn't mean the patient is fine. ERCP-based sampling, though helpful when positive, is notoriously insensitive. Brushings have a sensitivity hovering around 40%-45%, and forceps biopsies are only modestly better.[42] Combine them, and the yield improves, but not enough to silence your clinical suspicion when the rest of the case smells like cancer.

> If you're dealing with a biliary stricture and ERCP brushings are negative, don't relax just yet

So, what now? According to the ACG guideline, the best next step is to enhance your sampling approach during ERCP, preferably using multiple, complementary techniques. The days of a single brush pass are long gone. When faced with a persistent stricture, you should be thinking about:

- **Repeat brushings**
- **Forceps biopsies** (multiple, with aggressive technique)
- **FISH** (fluorescence in situ hybridization) to assess for chromosomal abnormalities in cytology specimens
- **Cholangioscopy-guided biopsies**, which allow for direct visualization and targeted sampling of suspicious mucosa.

Among these, direct cholangioscopy plays a key role. It has emerged as perhaps the most effective endoscopic tool for evaluating indeterminate strictures, especially when imaging and standard ERCP biopsies fall short. The guideline supports its use both for

Cholangioscopy may be the most effective endoscopic tool for evaluating indeterminate strictures

diagnostic purposes and targeted tissue acquisition. Studies show that visual impression alone during cholangioscopy has a sensitivity of about 90%—and when combined with biopsies, the diagnostic yield improves significantly.[43]

Chromosomal Clues: Making Sense of FISH Polysomy

Use of FISH can enhance detection of cancer. Look for polysomy, indicating extra chromosomal copies. PPV of polysomy is 80%

Brush cytology alone misses far too many cancers hiding inside dominant strictures, so we use FISH to light up chromosomal chaos the microscope can't see. The lab applies fluorescent probes to chromosomes 3, 7, 17, and the 9p21 locus. In a benign cell, you'll see 2 tidy signals per probe. In a cell that's gone rogue, you may see polysomy—3, 4, or a confetti storm of signals—indicating extra chromosomal copies and genomic instability, a red flag for cholangiocarcinoma.

Why do we care? In PSC (or any indeterminate biliary stricture), a single routine brushing is <40% sensitive, but if that same brushing shows polysomy on FISH, diagnostic yield jumps into the 60%-70% range and the positive predictive value for cancer can approach 80%, especially when polysomy is confirmed on 2 separate brushings.[44,45] In practical terms:

- **Polysomy + suspicious imaging** → fast-track to oncologic work-up or transplant center.
- **Polysomy once, then normal** → repeat ERCP with a second brushing; persistent polysomy is highly worrisome.
- **No polysomy, benign cytology, stable imaging** → you've bought follow-up time, but not a lifetime guarantee; keep the patient on a tight surveillance schedule with repeat imaging and, if doubt persists, cholangioscopy-directed biopsies.

Remember, FISH is an adjunct, not judge and jury. A positive result nudges the pre-test probability of malignancy way up; a negative result does not rule out cancer. Think of FISH polysomy as the ductal equivalent of a loud smoke alarm: you still have to find the fire, but you'd be crazy to ignore the noise.

Should you send this patient for EUS now? It depends. EUS has a high yield for sampling extrinsic compressions or pancreatic masses, but in the absence of a visible mass on MRCP or CT, the likelihood of a diagnostic EUS drops. That said, if there is any periductal soft tissue seen on imaging or suspicion of submucosal growth, EUS with FNA/FNB may still be helpful, especially if lymphadenopathy is present.

The key is to avoid redundancy. If the stricture is ductal and there's no adjacent mass, ERCP-based approaches (especially with cholangioscopy) usually also provide better intraductal access than EUS.

Now, let's say you've done it all — repeat ERCP with brushings and biopsies, FISH, cholangioscopy, and perhaps even EUS — and still, no definitive answer. At this point, you're in management limbo: there's a persistent stricture, high clinical suspicion, but no tissue confirmation.

The guideline advises that persistent indeterminate strictures after multimodal sampling should be discussed in a multidisciplinary tumor board. This isn't a punt — it's a strategy. Some of these cases may warrant surgical exploration despite the absence of positive cytology, particularly if the pre-test probability of cancer is high and the stricture is surgically accessible.

Persistent biliary stricture despite bunch of work-up? Discuss the case in a multidisciplinary tumor board

In the case presented, where the patient is symptomatic and imaging shows a tight mid-CBD stricture with negative brushings, the next best step would be a repeat ERCP with cholangioscopy-directed biopsies, and consideration of FISH analysis if cytology remains equivocal. EUS could be considered if imaging reveals periductal changes or lymph nodes. And if it all remains inconclusive, a tumor board should weigh in on whether to proceed to surgical exploration or repeat sampling in expert hands.

Bringing It Together

When it comes to indeterminate biliary strictures, a single ERCP with negative brushings isn't the end of the road — it's just the beginning. The guideline emphasizes a multimodal, layered diagnostic approach, incorporating cholangioscopy, FISH, and (in selected cases) EUS.

Don't rely on 1 technique to carry the whole diagnostic weight — stack them. And if you've done everything right and still don't have an answer, don't freeze. Get a tumor board involved, and consider referring for surgical exploration if the clinical picture keeps pointing toward malignancy.

To summarize this vignette, check out **Table 2.2**, which describes the strengths, limitations, and ideal use cases of different diagnostic tools for managing indeterminate biliary strictures.

Table 2.2. *Diagnostic Tools for Indeterminate Biliary Strictures.*

Diagnostic tool	Role/Strengths	Limitations	Ideal Use Case
Brush cytology (ERCP)	Widely available; easy to perform	Low sensitivity (~45%); nonspecific atypia common	Initial ERCP sampling; combine with other methods
Forceps biopsy (ERCP)	Higher yield than brushings when multiple samples taken	Technically challenging; limited reach	Tight strictures; best when combined with brushings
FISH analysis	Detects chromosomal changes (e.g., polysomy)	Not definitive for cancer; adds cost	PSC patients; equivocal cytology
Cholangioscopy	Direct visualization; targeted biopsies; ~90% visual sensitivity	Requires expertise and equipment; costly	Persistent strictures with negative sampling
EUS-FNA/FNB	High yield for extrinsic masses or lymph nodes	Lower yield for purely intraductal lesions	Visible mass, lymphadenopathy, periductal thickening
Tumor board discussion	Multidisciplinary input; surgical planning	Doesn't provide tissue; may delay decisions	After negative multimodal workup

Case 2.3: Steel Curtain Defense

A 45-year-old man with a long history of alcohol-related chronic pancreatitis presents with worsening fatigue, pale stools, and scleral icterus. He's had 2 hospitalizations in the past year for acute-on-chronic pancreatitis flares, but has been abstinent from alcohol for the past 6 months.

Labs show a total bilirubin of 4.8 mg/dL, ALP of 410 U/L, and mildly elevated transaminases. CA 19-9 is 24 U/mL.

MRCP reveals a high-grade distal common bile duct stricture with upstream intrahepatic biliary dilation. There is no discrete mass, and pancreatic calcifications and ductal changes consistent with chronic pancreatitis are noted. He undergoes ERCP with brushings and forceps biopsies, which return negative for malignancy. EUS shows no mass or lymphadenopathy. His symptoms improve after placement of a 10 Fr plastic biliary stent.

The plan is to repeat ERCP in 3 months. The patient asks: *How long will I need this stent?*

Know your guidelines!

1. How are benign biliary strictures diagnosed and distinguished from malignant ones?
2. What is the optimal stenting strategy for benign strictures — plastic vs metal?
3. How long should therapy last, and how will you define success?
4. Are there special considerations in chronic pancreatitis compared to post-surgical or autoimmune strictures?

Case 2.3: What do the guidelines say?

Source: ACG 2023 Management of Biliary Strictures Guidelines[39]

> Malignant strictures seldom stay quiet after 3-6 months of close observation

Benign biliary strictures love to masquerade as malignancy. In chronic pancreatitis, long-standing inflammation, periductal fibrosis, calcifications, and scarring can narrow the distal CBD so convincingly that even high-resolution MRI begs for a second opinion. A normal or only mildly elevated CA 19-9 (as in this patient) is reassuring, but as we've seen in an earlier vignette, never diagnostic. What ultimately seals the deal is negative multimodal sampling plus compatible imaging and, just as importantly, time: malignant strictures seldom stay quiet after 3 to 6 months of close observation. In this case the patient has had brushings, forceps biopsies, and EUS with no red flags for cancer; the stricture therefore falls squarely into the "benign—most likely inflammatory" bucket.

Choose Your Hardware Wisely: Multiple Plastics or a Fully-Covered SEMS?

> Treat benign strictures with fcSEMS over parallel plastic stents, provided the cystic duct isn't covered

Once malignancy is off the table, the conversation shifts from "Is it cancer?" to "How do we keep the duct open long-term?" The ACG guideline recommends using a fully-covered self-expanding metal stents (fcSEMS) over parallel plastic stents for most benign extrahepatic strictures — provided the cystic duct orifice isn't covered (to avoid cholecystitis). In essence, the fcSEMS provides a steel curtain defense to maintain patency and is the best option. Kinda how the impenetrable "Steel Curtain" defense enabled the greatest NFL franchise, the illustrious Pittsburgh Steelers, to become 6-time Super Bowl champions. At any rate, there are several benefits of fcSEMSs, including:

- Larger diameter and radial force → faster dilation
- Fewer ERCP sessions (often just 2: placement and removal)
- Comparable or better long-term success than the traditional "stent-packing" strategy of 4 to 6 plastic stents exchanged every 3 months.

Parallel plastic stents still have a role when the cystic duct is at risk, in post liver transplant anastomotic strictures (where the tortuosity can trap a metal stent), or when local expertise with metal stent removal is limited.

How Long Is Long Enough?

For benign strictures treated with multiple plastics, the rule of thumb is 12 months of dwell time, exchanging and upsizing every 3 months. Metal stent therapy is at minimum 6 months of dwelling, although many experts push to 12 months because the recurrence rates fall when the fcSEMS stay in longer. If you aim for the full year, the guideline suggests a midway fcSEMS exchange to prevent embedment. In chronic pancreatitis strictures, success (defined as a patent duct 6 months after stent removal) runs about 90% with metal stents, which work just as well as plastic stents but require fewer exchanges.[46-48]

> In general, best to keep stents in for 12 months to treat benign strictures, with exchanges every 3 months for plastic, and at 6 months for fcSEMS

Special Wrinkles in Chronic Pancreatitis

- **Calcified, rigid ducts**: They can grip a metal stent like concrete. Meticulous sleeve removal technique (dilation, grasping forceps, sometimes cholangioscopic guidance) lowers the risk of embedding.
- **High recurrence risk**: Smoking, ongoing alcohol use, and poorly controlled diabetes worsen fibrosis and raise relapse rates. Strict lifestyle counseling is part of the therapy, not an adjunct.
- **Adjunctive therapy**: Pancreatic duct stenting or ESWL (lithotripsy) to clear intraductal stones may indirectly relieve biliary compression.

Bringing It Together

Benign doesn't mean easy. First, prove it's benign with thorough, multimodal sampling and vigilant follow-up. Then choose the stent that maximizes duct caliber while minimizing ERCP fatigue: fcSEMS if anatomy allows, parallel plastics when it doesn't. Leave metal in for at least 6 months (and preferably 12, with a midpoint swap), coach the patient hard on alcohol abstinence and smoking cessation, and check liver tests at each waypoint. When the stent finally comes out and the bilirubin stays low 6 months later, you—and the patient's beleaguered bile duct—can finally exhale. See **Table 2.3** for a summary of this vignette.

Table 2.3. *Stent strategy for benign extrahepatic strictures.*

Strategy	Typical dwell time	ERCP sessions	Pros	Cons
Multiple plastic stents (4-6 in parallel)	~12 mo (exhcange/ upsizing q3 mo)	4-5	Familiar, inexpensive hardware	More procedures, lower diameters
fcSEMS	>6 mo (ideally 12 mo; mid-exchange at 6 mo)	2-3	Larger caliber, fewer ERCPs, higher one-and-done success	Risk of cystic-duct obstruction; extraction can be tricky
Uncovered SEMS	Avoid in benign disease	—	—	Tissue ingrowth; non-removable

Case 2.4: Danger at the Crossing

A 65-year-old woman is referred for evaluation of a new perihilar biliary stricture discovered during workup for fatigue and mild pruritus. Her labs show a total bilirubin of 3.6 mg/dL, elevated alkaline phosphatase, and mild transaminemia. CA 19-9 is 140 U/mL.

She has no history of liver disease, IBD, or autoimmune conditions. An MRCP reveals a dominant hilar stricture involving the hepatic duct confluence with upstream intrahepatic biliary dilation (**Figure 2.2**). There is no discrete mass. A subsequent ERCP confirms the stricture, and brushings are non-diagnostic. The patient is referred to your center for further evaluation.

Figure 2.2. *MRCP with hilar stricture noted by non-visualization of the confluence of the right and left hepatic ducts with upstream biliary dilation.*[49]

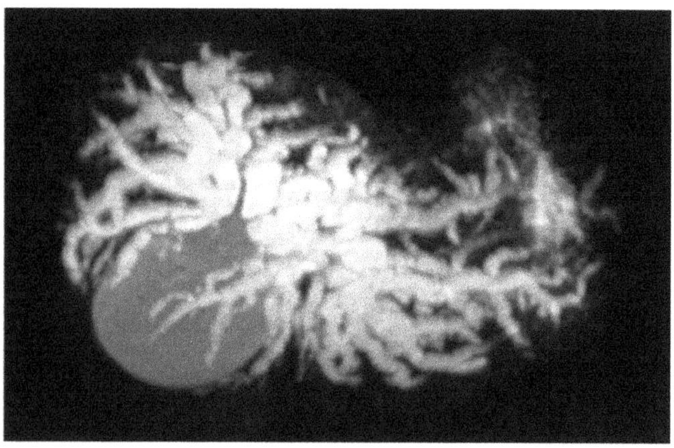

Know your guidelines!

1. What is the differential diagnosis for a hilar stricture?
2. What are the preferred methods for tissue acquisition in perihilar strictures?
3. Should you FNA/FNB the lesion directly with EUS?
4. What's the role of node sampling — and how does transplant candidacy affect this?
5. When do you drain, and how do you avoid worsening the situation?

Case 2.4: What do the guidelines say?

Source: ACG 2023 Management of Biliary Strictures Guidelines[39]

A solitary, high-grade stricture at the hepatic duct confluence makes cholangiocarcinoma the odds-on favorite, but the differential is broader than some realize. Perihilar narrowing can also arise from metastatic nodes, IgG4-related sclerosing cholangitis, postpartum biliary injury, ischemia after liver transplantation, or (in a PSC patient), an inflammatory "dominant stricture." Yet statistics are merciless: in a large surgical series, about 85% of isolated hilar strictures turned out to be malignant.[50,51] The CA 19-9 of 140 U/mL in this case supports—without confirming—the malignant hunch.

Sampling Strategy: Keep your needle out of the hilum

The ACG guideline draws a bright line here: intraductal sampling at ERCP (brushings ± forceps ± FISH ± cholangioscopy) is preferred over EUS-FNA/FNB of the primary hilar lesion. Direct needle puncture risks tumor seeding along the needle tract, which could be disastrous if transplant is on the table.[52] So if there is a doubt on transplant eligibility, hold on doing an EUS until you talk to your transplant center and review their protocols. Even though EUS can sample regional portocaval and periportal lymph nodes, staging is typically done by imaging before neoadjuvant therapy within cholangiocarcinoma protocols.

> For a hilar lesion, go to ERCP (preferably with cholangioscopy, if available)

Check out **Table 2.4** for a handy review of different tissue-acquisition approaches for suspected hilar cholangiocarcinoma.

Drain, But Only When You Help—Never When You Harm

When draining a perihilar stricture, the goal isn't to fill every duct with a stent — it's to relieve obstruction in enough of the liver to make a clinical difference. The European guideline also emphasizes that draining at least 50% of the functional liver volume is typically sufficient to lower bilirubin, improve symptoms, and enable chemotherapy when indicated.[53] Cross-sectional imaging (CT or

Table 2.4. *Tissue-Acquistion Roadmap for Suspected Hilar Cancer.*

Target	Allowed?	Rational/Caveat
Intraductal brushings (ERCP)	Yes	Easy, safe, but low sensitivity —combine with other tools
Forceps biopsies (ERCP)	Yes	Adds yield; take multiple passes
FISH on cytology	Yes	Detects polysomy; helpful when brushings are "atypical"
Cholangioscopy-directed biopsies	Yes	Highest intraductal yield; needs expertise
EUS-FNA/FNB	No, unless not a transplant candidate	Risk of peritoneal seeding; can preclude transplantation

MRI) should guide which ducts you target — ideally those supplying the largest, most functional segments of the liver.

Trying to drain too many segments can backfire, especially in higher Bismuth-Corlette types — a classification system for perihilar cholangiocarcinomas based on how far the tumor extends into the left and right hepatic ducts. Types III and IV involve both sides of the biliary tree and create complex anatomy that makes full drainage difficult or risky. In these cases, aggressive stenting can increase the risk of cholangitis from undrained segments or lead to technical failure. So be selective: drain what matters, not everything in sight. **Figure 2.3** provides a breakdown of the Bismuth-Corlette classification system.

Figure 2.3. *Bismuth-Corlette classification system of perihilar cholangiocarcinomas. The yellow or purple areas represent tumor locations and the green areas are normal.*[54]

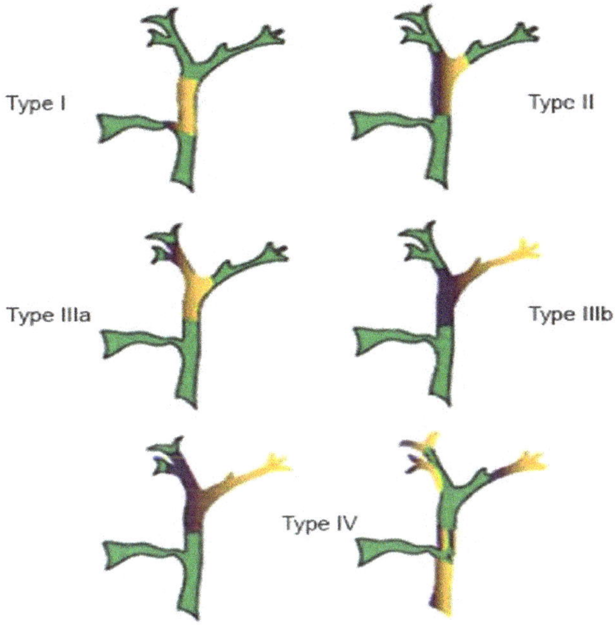

Teaching Points

- Skip the heroic EUS needle pass through the hilum; you may cure your curiosity but kill a transplant option.
- Load up on intraductal sampling at the next ERCP—brush, bite, maybe cholangioscopy, send for FISH.
- Drain only the segments that matter.

Bottom line: Perihilar strictures demand procedural discipline. Diagnose intraductally and only puncture the hilum or nodes when cure is no longer in play. Respect that rule to keep surgical and transplant doors open while steering the patient toward the right therapy at the right time.

Case 2.5: A Stent Too Soon?

A 69-year-old man is diagnosed with pancreatic head adenocarcinoma after presenting with mild epigastric discomfort, early satiety, and unintentional weight loss. Cross-sectional imaging reveals a 2.5-cm mass in the pancreatic head, without vascular involvement and without metastasis. His CA 19-9 is 310 U/mL.

A referring GI physician performs ERCP and places a 7 Fr plastic biliary stent due to an elevated bilirubin of 6.5 mg/dL and mild pruritus. The plan is for Whipple resection in 1 week.

He now presents to your center for surgical evaluation. The surgeon expresses concern about the stent, *We would've preferred to operate on native ducts*. Meanwhile, the bilirubin is trending down.

Know your guidelines!

1. Should patients with resectable pancreatic cancer receive routine preoperative biliary drainage?
2. If drainage is necessary, what type of stent is preferred?
3. What are the risks of early stenting — and when is it appropriate?
4. Does a plastic stent suffice if surgery is imminent?

Case 2.5: What do the guidelines say?

Source: ACG 2023 Management of Biliary Strictures Guidelines[39]

For resectable pancreatic head cancer, the ACG guideline specifically advises against routine biliary drainage. Why? Pre-op stenting adds a second procedure, invites cholangitis or pancreatitis, often clogs before surgery, and can contaminate an otherwise pristine operative field. Trials comparing "straight to knife" versus "stent then knife" show higher infection and surgical delay rates in the stented cohort, with no survival benefit.[41] The only clear winners are endoscopists and supply reps.

Planning surgery for pancreatic head cancer? Avoid pre-op stenting unless absolutely necessary

But When Does Drainage Make Sense?

For pre-op stenting, the guideline carves out a short, sensible list, which we covered in an earlier vignette but it bears repeating here:

- Acute cholangitis
- Severe, sleep-stealing pruritus
- "Very high" bilirubin (about 15+)
- Anticipated delay to surgery (neoadjuvant therapy, cardiac workup, bed shortage, need to improve nutritional status, etc.)

Our patient had modest pruritus and a bilirubin of 6.5 mg/dL, with a 1-week path to the OR—solidly in the "no stent needed" zone.

If you must drain, choose the right tubing.

Plastic stents are cheap and quick, which is why some centers may love them. Alas, they occlude in weeks, slime the duct with biofilm, and demand another ERCP when the surgeon least wants one. The guideline favors a self-expanding metal stent (SEMS) whenever drainage is truly necessary in potentially resectable disease, since SEMS:

- Expand to 8-10 mm, clearing jaundice fast
- Resist clogging for months (handy if neoadjuvant therapy appears)
- Can be removed at surgery—or endoscopically if plans change.

Now what about the plastic already in place?

Fortunately, a single 7 Fr plastic stent left in for <2 weeks rarely derails a Whipple. However, if a plastic stent is chosen, then it would have been more prudent to go with a bigger diameter (like 10 Fr) to reduce the risk of occlusion.[55] Discuss with the surgeon: many will proceed without exchange, removing the stent en bloc during resection. If bilirubin remains stubbornly high, an interval ERCP to swap plastics for an SEMS can still salvage patency—but only if it won't delay the OR date.

Bottom line: Pre-emptive drainage feels proactive but often backfires. Skip it unless the guideline's red flag indications are met. When you do drain, think first about placing a SEMS before you reach for the plastic. That single decision spares the patient extra ERCPs, can shield the surgeon from cholangitic surprise, and keeps the path clear for cure.

Case 2.6: The Narrowing Path

A 42-year-old man with a 5-year history of primary sclerosing cholangitis (PSC) presents with new onset fatigue, worsening pruritus, and mild right upper quadrant discomfort. He does not report fever, jaundice, or weight loss. His labs show a total bilirubin of 3.2 mg/dL, alkaline phosphatase of 490 U/L, and mildly elevated AST and ALT.

An MRCP reveals multifocal intrahepatic stricturing and a new 1.3-mm dominant stricture in the common bile duct without significant upstream dilation and no change in left-sided intrahepatic biliary beading (arrows in **Figure 2.4**). He has no prior history of cholangitis. Serum CA 19-9 is 88 U/mL. A recent colonoscopy confirmed quiescent ulcerative pancolitis.

Figure 2.4. *Dominant Stricture on MRCP in Patient with PSC.*[56]

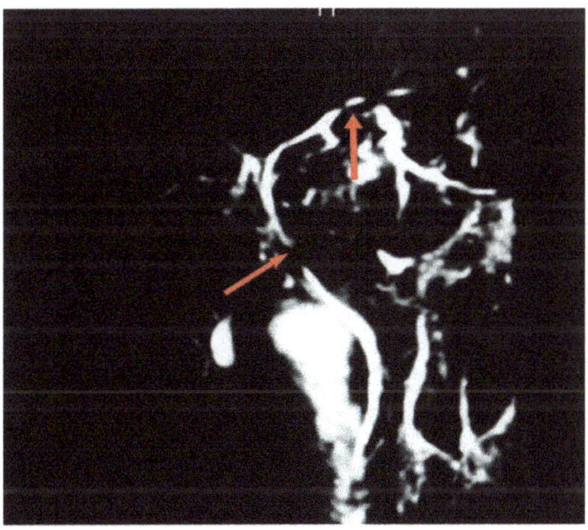

The patient is referred for ERCP to evaluate the new stricture.

Know your guidelines!

1. How do you define a dominant stricture in PSC?
2. What's the role of ERCP in evaluating and treating these strictures?
3. Should you place a stent — or stick with balloon dilation?
4. How do you assess for cholangiocarcinoma?
5. When does a dominant stricture signal something worse?

Case 2.6: What do the guidelines say?

Source: ACG 2015 Primary Sclerosing Cholangitis Guidelines[57]

In PSC it is easy to become blasé about narrow ducts—until one of them crosses the line from "background noise" to a dominant stricture (DS). By convention, a DS is a focal narrowing of the common hepatic duct to < 1.5 mm or of a right or left hepatic duct to < 1 mm on cholangiography.[58] Strictures this tight obstruct bile flow, drive bilirubin upward, provoke pruritus and cholangitis, and—most importantly—harbor or herald cholangiocarcinoma (CCA). In short, a DS is the moment in PSC when vigilance and intervention genuinely change a patient's trajectory.

In PSC, a dominant stricture means common hepatic duct <1.5 mm or right or left hepatic ducts <1 mm

Step 1: Is this cancer in disguise?

Before anything is dilated or stented, the endoscopist must supply tissue to the pathologist—because clinical clues rarely clinch the diagnosis. Serum CA 19-9, for instance, is a helpful compass (levels > 129 U/mL increase the odds of CCA several-fold), yet it misleads often enough that treatment decisions cannot rest on the number alone, as we've seen from previous vignettes. Cross-sectional imaging gives a map of biliary anatomy and flags overt masses, but half of CCAs at the hilum are still radiologically occult.

The real work therefore occurs at ERCP. Interventionalists typically make 1 controlled balloon inflation (just enough to let accessories pass) and then obtain samples in 3 complementary ways, shown in **Table 2.5.**

Table 2.5. *"Triple-Play" Diagnostic Sampling for a PSC Dominant Stricture.*

Modality	Why it matters	Typical yield
Brush cytology	Fast, cheap, universally available	~40% sensitivity
Forceps biopsies	Adds architecture and DNA	Bumps sensitivity to 50%-55%
FISH for chromosomal polysomy	Detects malignant clones even when morphology looks bland	Lifts overall sensitivity to ≥60%

When conventional tools remain inconclusive, yet suspicion persists, single-operator cholangioscopy lets us target the most ominous surface for biopsy and can push sensitivity to about 90%.[59] Moreover, cholangioscopy can help find bile duct stones missed on cholangiography.[60] EUS-guided sampling is not recommended if the patient is a potential liver transplant candidate under a cholangiocarcinoma protocol due to the real risk of transperitoneal needle track seeding; thus, sabotaging future transplant eligibility.[52]

Step 2: Open the bottleneck

Once malignancy has been reasonably excluded (or at least sampled), the same session turns therapeutic. For most dominant strictures, endoscopic balloon dilation alone is the ACG-endorsed strategy. A high-pressure 6-10 mm balloon held for 60-120 seconds usually suffices; the visual cue of a disappearing waist followed by a gush of contrast back toward the duodenum is immensely satisfying. Routine stenting, by contrast, adds little benefit and a good deal of risk: plastic tubes clog, incubate bacteria, and drag patients back for early repeat ERCP. Stents are kept in reserve for the rare stricture that recoils immediately or for palliative decompression when proven CCA obstructs the hilum.

Endoscopic balloon dilation is usually first-line therapy for a DS in PSC

Because bile is already sluggish in PSC, every therapeutic ERCP occurs under the shadow of post-procedure cholangitis.[61] Periprocedural antibiotics are mandatory, and continued for several days if contrast drainage during the case is incomplete. When infection does complicate a DS, it can be formidable—prompt recognition and low thresholds for repeat ERCP or percutaneous drainage save lives. Interestingly enough, statins not only have a beneficial effect on metabolic disease-related outcomes, but have also been shown to decrease the risk of cholangitis in PSC by 81%. This seems to be related to their propensity to lengthen the time for dominant stricture formation.[62] Moreover, statin use in PSC patients has been associated with decreased mortality and liver transplantation.[63]

Just...wow!

Step 3: Make sure the fix sticks

Most patients feel better within days: bilirubin drifts downward, pruritus eases, and appetite returns. Consider repeating liver chemistries at 4-6 weeks; if bilirubin remains >3 mg/dL or symptoms relapse, another look is warranted. In the absence of red flags, you can shift into surveillance mode: yearly MRCP coupled with CA 19-9 monitoring keeps a watchful eye for CCA and for new strictures that will eventually need the same drill.

Why This Matters

Ballooning a DS is more than a technical flourish: it delays cirrhosis by restoring bile flow, slashes hospitalizations for cholangitis, and, has been associated with better transplant-free survival.[64-66] Equally important, meticulous sampling at the first encounter can catch a CCA early enough for curative resection or for entry into transplant-based protocols.

Bottom line: A dominant stricture is PSC's wolf in sheep's clothing. Treat it as malignant until multiple sampling modalities say otherwise; use balloon dilation as your therapeutic mainstay; and never skimp on antibiotics or follow-up imaging. Mastering that sequence keeps the road open for transplantation and spares patients the misery of unchecked obstruction—and that is a victory worth the fluoroscopy time.

Case 2.7: PSC's Silent Partner

A 39-year-old woman is referred for evaluation of abnormal liver tests discovered during routine blood work. She feels entirely well and has not experienced abdominal pain, diarrhea, rectal bleeding, weight loss, or fatigue. Labs show: ALP 412 U/L; AST 52 U/L; ALT 58 U/L; total bilirubin 1.1 mg/dL; albumin 4.2 g/dL; international normalized ratio (INR) 1.0. MRCP reveals multifocal intrahepatic and extrahepatic bile duct stricturing with saccular dilatations, like a "chain of lakes," shown in **Figure 2.5.** She has never had a colonoscopy.

Figure 2.5. *"Chain of Lakes" on MRCP.*[67]

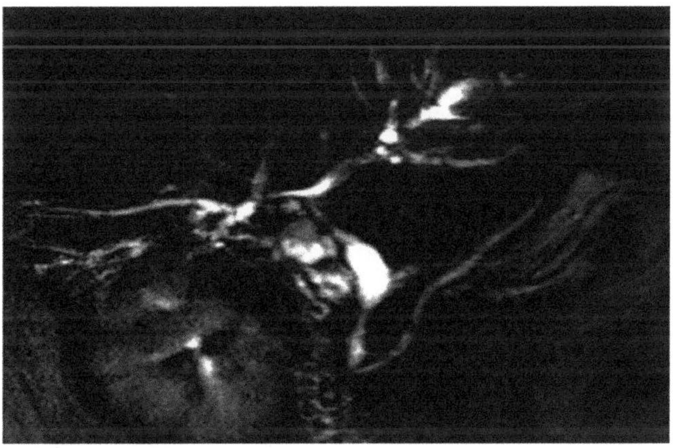

Know your guidelines!

1. Should this patient get a colonoscopy, even if asymptomatic?
2. How does PSC-associated IBD differ from typical ulcerative colitis or Crohn's disease?
3. What surveillance strategy is recommended if colitis is confirmed?
4. Should chromoendoscopy be used for dysplasia surveillance in PSC?
5. What are the implications of silent pancolitis on long-term management and cancer risk?

Case 2.7: What do the guidelines say?

Source: ACG 2015 Primary Sclerosing Cholangitis Guidelines[57]

When a newly diagnosed PSC patient tells you they feel fine, they usually mean it. In fact, many will have completely silent disease—no jaundice, no cholangitis, no weight loss, no symptoms of any kind. But what's deceptive is that the colon can be quietly involved too, and that changes everything.

All patients with newly diagnosed PSC should get a colonoscopy, even if asymptomatic

The ACG guideline recommend that all patients with newly diagnosed PSC undergo a full colonoscopy with biopsies at the time of diagnosis, regardless of whether they report any GI symptoms or whether they are old enough for colorectal cancer screening. This is not a reflexive overreach — it's a strategic move based on decades of clinical observation: most patients with PSC have underlying inflammatory bowel disease (IBD), and much of it flies under the radar. In fact, the prevalence of IBD in PSC is as high as 80%, and a substantial number of those patients are asymptomatic at diagnosis. The colonic mucosa may look deceptively normal on endoscopy, which is why random biopsies are essential, even when the mucosa looks clean.

Up to 80% of patients with PSC have underlying IBD

PSC-IBD Is Its Own Animal

The combination of PSC and IBD is a different beast than either condition alone. Patients with PSC-associated colitis have a significantly elevated risk of colorectal cancer, estimated at 4- to 5-fold higher than patients with IBD without PSC. The disease also has a distinct phenotype: right-sided predominance, rectal sparing, and frequent quiescence, even in the setting of histologic inflammation. This means you can't rely on symptoms, and you can't wait for bleeding or diarrhea to tell you when to investigate.

PSC-related IBD has 4-5 x risk of colon cancer compared to IBD alone

Surveillance Starts Now

Once colitis is confirmed, the clock starts on surveillance. The guideline recommends annual colonoscopy with chromoendoscopy (if available) for dysplasia detection. This differs markedly from standard IBD surveillance intervals, which typically begin 8 years after diagnosis and continue every 1-3 years. In PSC, you start now, and you stay vigilant. Even if the patient is asymptomatic, and even if the colitis is histologically mild, the risk of colorectal neoplasia is persistent and real.[68] It's even more imperative for patients with indefinite or low-grade dysplasia to be tightly monitored with colonoscopy and tissue samples reviewed by expert GI pathologists.

In PSC with IBD, begin annual colonoscopy upon diagnosis and use chromoendoscopy if available

It's also worth noting that finding IBD may influence other aspects of care, including eligibility and timing for liver transplant. In some cases, the presence of PSC-IBD informs the choice of immunosuppressants post-transplant and guides decisions around colectomy, particularly if dysplasia emerges. Of course, don't forget that an ERCP is still needed for further evaluation due to that dominant stricture in the mid-common bile duct (take another look at that MRCP image in **Figure 2.6**).

Bottom line: Every patient with newly diagnosed PSC deserves a baseline colonoscopy with biopsies—whether they feel fine or not. Most will have silent IBD, often pancolitis, and that dramatically alters their colorectal cancer risk and surveillance schedule. Symptoms may lie, but the histology won't—and early detection is the only way to stay ahead of PSC's quiet accomplice.

Case 2.8: Not So Fast...

A 20-year-old man is referred for evaluation of elevated ALP discovered during workup for fatigue. Labs show: ALP 602 U/L; AST 126 U/L; ALT 134 U/L; total bilirubin 1.2 mg/dL. He does not report pruritus, jaundice, or weight loss. His antinuclear antibody (ANA) and anti-smooth muscle antibody (ASMA) are negative, but his total serum IgG is mildly elevated at 2,100 mg/dL. MRCP shows multifocal intrahepatic bile duct stricturing and mild ductal dilatation, raising concern for PSC.

The outside referring GI notes a "probable PSC diagnosis," but the hepatologist reviewing the case pauses. "He's 20. Something's not adding up here..."

Know your guidelines!

1. What are the key mimickers of PSC, and how do you distinguish them?
2. When should you check serum IgG4 — and what does an elevated result suggest?
3. Who needs a liver biopsy, and what are the classic histologic findings?
4. What clinical scenarios should trigger evaluation for autoimmune hepatitis overlap?

Case 2.8: What do the guidelines say?

Source: ACG 2015 Primary Sclerosing Cholangitis Guidelines[57]

A multifocal biliary stricture pattern on MRCP invites a reflex diagnosis of PSC. In a 20-year-old, however, the warning light on your diagnostic dashboard should blink, "**Confirm before committing!**" Classic PSC certainly occurs in young adults, but mimickers and overlaps become proportionally more common as age drops. Failure to separate them from PSC is more than a nomenclature error—it forfeits therapies that can halt progression or even reverse disease.

The Cholangitic Impostors

At the top of the rule-out list are IgG4-related sclerosing cholangitis (IgG4-SC), autoimmune hepatitis (AIH) overlap, and a basket of secondary sclerosing cholangitides (ischemia, infection, postsurgical injury, toxins). Each can masquerade as PSC on imaging, yet each has its own treatment path. **Table 2.6** outlines the differential diagnosis of PSC, IgG4-SC, AIH-PSC overlap, and secondary SC examples.

PSC mimics include:

* IgG4 scerlosing cholangitis
* AIH-PSC overlap
* Ischemia
* Chronic biliary infection
* Postsurgical injury

Laboratory Triage—Don't Skip the IgG4

Guidelines advise checking serum IgG4 at least once in every PSC evaluation; an elevation (>135 mg/dL, or >2× ULN for stronger specificity) should prompt an IgG4-centric work-up, including pancreas and salivary imaging. While this patient's total IgG is mildly high, an isolated hyper-γ-globulinemia often flags AIH overlap—another reason to dig deeper rather than brand him PSC and move on. We need to check the IgG4 subclass, not just total IgG.

When to Reach for the Biopsy Needle

A liver biopsy is not required for classic PSC, but his profile triggers two guideline-supported biopsy indications: age <25 years and aminotransferases disproportionately high (AST/ALT roughly 5 times ULN). The core aims are:

Table 2.6. *The PSC Imposters.*
AIH, autoimmune hepatitis; ANA, antinuclear antibody; PSC, primary sclerosing cholangitis; SMA, smooth muscle antibody; ULN, upper limit normal.

Feature	Classic PSC	IgG4-SC	AIH-PSC overlap	Secondary SC (selected examples)
Typical age/sex	30-50 yr, male > female	>50 yr, male predominance but younger cases occur	<30 yr, any sex	Variable; depends on cause
Serum IGg4	Usually normal	Often >135 mg/dL (may be mildly elevated)	Normal or mild↑	Normal
Aminotransferases	Mild-mod↑	Mild↑	Often ≥5 x ULN	Variable; may spike in acute insults
Histology	Periductal "onion-skin" fibrosis	Storiform fibrosis, obliterative phlebitis, IgG4 plasma cells (>10/HPF)	Interface hepatitis, plasma cell rich infiltrate	Depends on etiology (ischemic concentric fibrosis, neutrophilic cholangitis, etc)
Immunologic clues	p-ANCA+/-	Other organ IgG4 disease (pancreas, salivary glands)	ANA or SMA positive in ~70%	Usually seronegative
First-line therapy	Endoscopic palliation; eventually transplant	Glucocorticoids ± rituximab, often dramatic response	Glucocorticoids → AZA/MMF	Treat underlying cause (antibiotics, revascularization, ERCP)

1. Look for interface hepatitis or plasma cell infiltrates pointing to AIH.
2. Quantify IgG4-positive plasma cells (>10 per high-power field strongly suggests IgG4-SC).
3. Exclude other patterns—ischemic concentric fibrosis, suppurative cholangitis—that would redirect therapy.

Biopsy also gives baseline fibrosis staging—a useful prognostic anchor no matter what name the disease finally carries. **Figure 2.6** shows a representative photomicrograph of lymphoplasmacytic portal infiltrates with duct injury and inflammation in our patient with "probable" PSC, indicating likely PSC-AIH overlap.

Figure 2.6. *PSC-AIH Overlap with duct injury and inflammation with lymphoplasmacytic portal infiltrate.*[69]

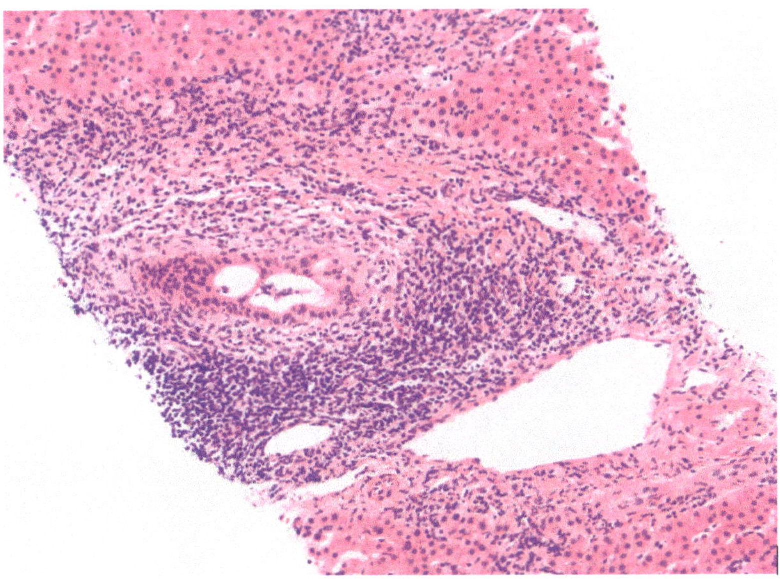

Clinical Stakes of a Correct Label

If this is IgG4-SC, a short steroid taper can normalize biochemistry in weeks and forestall biliary scarring. If it's AIH overlap, lifelong immunosuppression may be indicated; if untreated, overlap progresses more rapidly to cirrhosis than PSC alone. Even secondary etiologies such as recurrent bacterial cholangitis mandate antibiotic and endoscopic strategies very different from PSC surveillance. In other words, a mislabel isn't benign—it denies the patient the most effective, sometimes curative, interventions.

Bringing It Together

For our 20-year-old, the smart diagnostic sequence is:

1. Check serum IgG4 (and total IgG subclasses).
2. Order autoimmune serologies—ANA, SMA, IgG level.
3. Schedule a liver biopsy to hunt for AIH interface activity, IgG4-rich infiltrates, or secondary patterns.
4. Keep secondary cholangitis clues (trauma, ischemia, infection) on the radar and, if suggested, pursue targeted imaging or ERCP with brushings.

If IgG4-SC or AIH overlap is confirmed, initiate steroids (± azathioprine/mycophenolate mofetil) and monitor response. If biopsy and serology show classic PSC, manage per standard algorithms—but now with confidence the right door has been chosen.

Bottom line: PSC is a diagnosis of exclusion. In a patient under 25—or any patient who doesn't read like the PSC textbook—slow down and interrogate the imitators.

Case 2.9: Stricture on the Edge

A 48-year-old man with a 6-year history of PSC is rushed to the ED complaining of shaking chills, fever to 102°F, and a deep ache under his right ribs. Over the past month, he has also noticed darker urine, 2 daytime episodes of pruritus so intense he scratched until bleeding, and a 5-pound weight loss he blames on "no appetite."

Initial labs reveal: WBC 14.8 K/μL; total bilirubin 5.2 mg/dL; ALP 910 U/L; AST 128 U/L; ALT 112 U/L; INR 1.3; Creatinine 1.0 mg/dL. Blood cultures are drawn and broad-spectrum IV cefepime is started. Ultrasound shows mild intrahepatic ductal dilation but no stones; the gallbladder was removed 5 years ago. MRCP performed the next morning pinpoints a tight narrowing at the extrahepatic biliary confluence with upstream dilation, but no discrete mass.

He stabilizes with fluids and antibiotics, but by day 2, his itch and low-grade fever persist. The hepatology team debates next steps: *dilate now, stent now, simply sample, or wait until cultures clear?* Meanwhile, the patient asks why no one can say yet whether this might be cancer.

Know your guidelines!

1. What is the first-line therapy?
2. When should you add prophylactic or post procedure antibiotics?
3. If cultures remain positive or fevers recur, what imaging or interventions should follow?

Case 2.9: What do the guidelines say?

Source: ACG 2015 Primary Sclerosing Cholangitis Guidelines[57]

Unlike the afebrile patient in Case 2.6 with a dominant stricture, this patient arrives shaking, febrile, and jaundiced. The immediate sequence is broad-spectrum IV antibiotics and fluids, blood cultures, and once hemodynamics are steady, urgent ERCP for source control. Delay beyond 24 hours increases recurrent sepsis and mortality risk.

How to Decompress in the Heat of Infection

With a tight extrahepatic dominant stricture, endoscopic drainage is preferred over percutaneous routes unless the anatomy is hostile. The debate is balloon dilation alone versus dilation followed by a stent.

- **Our bias**: start with balloon dilation of the stricture; reinject contrast and confirm free flow. If the waist persists or recoil is immediate, insert a stent with a plan for the patient to return in the short-term for removal to minimize stent-sepsis risk. (*Author B.S.* has never done an ERCP in his 25 years of GI practice, so he will just take this for granted; *Author H.K.* used to do ERCPs for many years but realized he needed a semblance of work-life balance, so he stopped long ago!)
- **Post-ERCP antibiotics**: ACG recommends 3-5 days of IV or high-bioavailability oral therapy after an ERCP performed in the setting of cholangitis, extending or narrowing once cultures return.

Should We Biopsy or Brush Today?

Sampling is not forbidden during an infected ERCP, but there are 2 practical issues:

Purulent nastiness in the duct can obscure dysplastic epithelium

1. **False-negatives abound** when bile is purulent; inflammation obscures dysplastic epithelium.
2. **Procedure time matters**—the longer we stay in, the higher the pancreatitis and cholangitis flare risk.

Most centers therefore perform minimal sampling in the urgent session—a single wide brush for cytology—then plan a second ERCP after sepsis and bilirubin fall, using the full multimodality arsenal with cholangioscopy (brush, forceps, FISH, etc.). That staged strategy respects both oncologic vigilance and acute-care pragmatism.

Reinfection = Early Transplant Referral

Despite a low Model for End-Stage Liver Disease (MELD) score of 11, recurrent or refractory cholangitis from dominant strictures can serve as a trigger for transplant evaluation and possible MELD exception points. Why? Because repeated sepsis drives morbidity, hospital days, and mortality out of proportion to the calculated score. One or two rewinds through the ED for chills and jaundice causing cholangitis and sepsis may justify liver transplant listing, particularly if serial dilations and/or stenting fail to keep the patient afebrile for the long term.

> No matter the MELD, recurrent or refractory cholangitis in PSC should trigger transplant evaluation

Monitoring After Drainage

- **Bilirubin should fall by ≥ 50% within a week;** failure implies residual obstruction or occult abscess.
- **Blood cultures** dictate antibiotic course length; persistent bacteremia after 48 hours → repeat imaging for collections.
- **Schedule the second-look ERCP at 6-8 weeks:** remove the stent, redilate if needed, perform full dysplasia/cancer sampling, and decide on long-term stent strategy or surgical consult.

> Expect bilirubin to fall by <50% within a week of stenting

Bottom line: In PSC, a dominant stricture plus cholangitis is a red alert scenario. Drain early, use short-term stent if balloon recoil persists, keep antibiotics running 3-5 days, and come back for deliberate cancer workup once the bile duct is quiet. Two strikes of cholangitis despite adequate endoscopic therapy move the patient towards the transplant runway—MELD score notwithstanding.

Case 2.10: A Little Polyp

A 51-year-old man with an 8-year history of PSC comes in for routine follow-up. He feels well overall and has no new symptoms. His most recent labs show stable liver tests: ALP 412 U/L; TB 1.5 mg/dL; AST 72 U/L; ALT 64 U/L.

An annual RUQ ultrasound, performed as part of routine surveillance, reveals a gallbladder polyp measuring 9 mm, with no associated gallstones, shadowing or wall thickening (**Figure 2.7**). His prior ultrasound 1 year ago showed no polyps or stones.

The radiologist recommends follow-up in 6 to 12 months. What say you?

Figure 2.7. *Gallbladder Polyp.*[70]

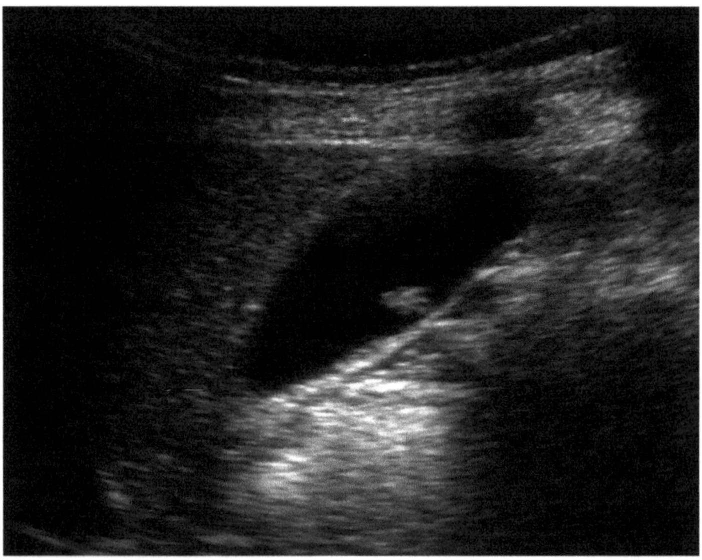

Know your guidelines!

1. How does polyp management differ in PSC vs the general population?
2. What is the cancer risk associated with gallbladder polyps in PSC?
3. What size threshold warrants referral for cholecystectomy?
4. Should surgery be performed even if the patient is asymptomatic?

Case 2.10: What do the guidelines say?

Source: ACG 2015 Primary Sclerosing Cholangitis Guidelines[57]

In PSC, the gallbladder is an "innocent bystander" only until it isn't: population studies show a 10- to 15-fold higher rate of gallbladder carcinoma compared with age-matched controls, and malignancy can arise even from small polyps.[71,72] For that reason, the ACG guideline directs us to obtain a screening right upper quadrant ultrasound every 12 months in every PSC patient, irrespective of symptoms or stage.

Do an RUQ U/S q12 months in PSC, even if no symptoms

Interpreting the 9-mm Polyp

Most gallbladder polyps in the general population are cholesterol polyps or adenomas with <1% malignant potential, so watch and wait is standard until they hit 10 mm. PSC rewrites that rule: histology series show that any polyp >8 mm (and occasionally even smaller ones) can harbor high-grade dysplasia or invasive adenocarcinoma; 1 Mayo cohort found adenocarcinoma in 14% of consecutive PSC patients who underwent liver transplant.[73] Size progression, wall thickening, or loss of the laminar "mucosa–submucosa" interface on ultrasound further raise suspicion.

GB polyp >8mm can mean trouble in PSC. Take it out, even if asymptomatic

Guideline-Driven Management

The ACG PSC guideline is unambiguous: **Cholecystectomy is recommended for gallbladder polyps >8 mm in PSC, even if asymptomatic.**

Because our patient's lesion measures 9 mm, the safest course is elective laparoscopic cholecystectomy in a center comfortable with portal hypertensive livers. If cirrhosis or significant varices pose a prohibitive risk, referral to transplant surgery for combined evaluation is prudent.

For completeness, smaller gallbladder polyps (≤8 mm) that are unequivocally benign-appearing need to be

In PSC, even very small GB polyps must be watched closely

watched very closely for any changes or symptoms. If there is any inkling of doubt, then bump the patient into the surgical lane.

Practical Pearls & Pitfalls

- Cross-sectional confirmation — if ultrasound is borderline or obscured by bowel gas, a quick MR or contrast CT helps nail exact size and exclude mural invasion.
- Portal vein pressures matter — pre-op endoscopy to stage varices and consider banding or beta blockade to reduce operative bleeding surprises.
- Patient counseling should stress that surgery is preventive: carcinoma can evolve rapidly with poor long-term survival after invasion.[74]

Bottom line: In PSC, a 9-mm gallbladder polyp is not a "wait and see" lesion—it is presumed premalignant until proven otherwise. Annual ultrasound caught it early; guideline-directed cholecystectomy now gives the patient the best shot at never meeting gallbladder cancer face-to-face.

Biliary Quiz

1. 1. A 62-year-old man with painless jaundice has a 2-cm mass in the pancreatic head and a distal CBD stricture. Which next step best aligns with ACG guidance?
   a. ERCP with plastic stent placement only
   b. EUS-FNA/FNB of the mass followed by ERCP in the same session
   c. Immediate surgical exploration without tissue diagnosis
   d. ERCP brush cytology first, postpone EUS until cytology result returns
   e. Place an uncovered metallic stent before oncology referral

2. During the ERCP portion of the above case, where the diagnosis is not yet known, which stent would be most appropriate if neoadjuvant chemotherapy is planned?
   a. 7 Fr plastic stent
   b. 10 Fr plastic stent
   c. Partially-covered SEMS
   d. Fully-covered SEMS
   e. Uncovered SEMS

3. Which factor independently favors EUS-guided sampling over ERCP sampling for extrahepatic strictures associated with a visible pancreatic mass?
   a. EUS has higher specificity
   b. ERCP carries higher risk of pancreatitis
   c. EUS has superior sensitivity for tissue diagnosis
   d. Brush cytology cannot be performed during ERCP
   e. EUS allows downstream stent placement

4. A 55-year-old woman has an indeterminate mid-CBD stricture after non-diagnostic brushings. Which adjunct improves diagnostic yield the most when added to repeat ERCP?
   a. Serum CA 19-9
   b. Percutaneous liver biopsy
   c. MRCP with secretin
   d. Serum CEA
   e. Cholangioscopy-directed biopsy

5. A 27-year-old man with established primary sclerosing cholangitis undergoes routine surveillance ultrasound. Imaging shows a single, sessile 5 mm gallbladder polyp with gallbladder wall thickening. His liver tests are unchanged from baseline. The best next step is:

   a. Immediate laparoscopic cholecystectomy
   b. Endoscopic polypectomy during ERCP
   c. Repeat right upper quadrant ultrasound in 6-12 months
   d. Begin high-dose ursodeoxycholic acid (28 mg/kg/day)
   e. MRI every 3 months until the polyp reaches 8 mm

6. A patient with chronic pancreatitis has a benign distal stricture requiring endoscopic therapy. The main advantage of a fully-covered SEMS over multiple plastic stents (MPS) is:

   a. Lower rate of migration
   b. Fewer ERCP sessions to achieve resolution
   c. Zero risk of pancreatitis
   d. No need for stent removal
   e. Lower cost of the stent itself

7. According to ACG, optimal duration of fcSEMS dwell time for benign CBD strictures is:

   a. <1 month
   b. 1-3 months
   c. ≥ 6 months
   d. Until symptoms recur
   e. Indefinitely

8. In a patient with gallbladder in situ whose cystic duct take-off will be covered by a metal stent, the guideline favors which stenting strategy for a biliary stricture?

   a. Multiple plastic stents instead of fcSEMS
   b. Uncovered SEMS
   c. Proceed with fcSEMS plus prophylactic cholecystectomy
   d. No stent; observe only
   e. Partially covered SEMS left permanently

9. A 68-year-old man has a Bismuth type IIIa hilar cholangiocarcinoma

deemed unresectable. Which initial drainage goal is guideline-concordant?

a. Drain only the left system
b. Drain ≥50 % of non-atrophic liver volume
c. Drain all sectors using uncovered SEMS in Y-configuration
d. Place single 7 Fr plastic stent across the hilum
e. Percutaneous biliary drainage of all ducts followed by ERCP stenting

10. In general, for most malignant hilar obstructions, which stent choice typically leads to longer patency?
    a. Single plastic stent
    b. Multiple plastic stents
    c. Uncovered SEMS
    d. Fully-covered SEMS
    e. Drug-eluting stent

11. Photodynamic therapy (PDT) is considered in PSC patients with unresectable cholangiocarcinoma primarily to:
    a. Cure the tumor
    b. Sterilize bile and prevent cholangitis
    c. Replace chemotherapy
    d. Reduce need for transplant evaluation
    e. Improve stent patency and quality of life

12. A 42-year-old man with PSC presents with worsening pruritus despite bile acid sequestrants. Of the choices listed below, what is the next best step?
    a. High-dose ursodeoxycholic acid 30 mg/kg/day
    b. Oral rifampin trial
    c. Liver transplantation listing solely for pruritus
    d. External biliary drain placement
    e. Plasmapheresis

13. What is the best strategy to confirm the diagnosis of small duct PSC?
    a. Liver biopsy
    b. MRCP
    c. ERCP
    d. EUS with FNA/FNB
    e. Serologic testing

14. In PSC, annual colonoscopy is recommended once colitis is confirmed because:

    a. Colorectal cancer risk is similar to sporadic polyps
    b. Risk of high-grade dysplasia is 4-5x higher than UC alone
    c. Colonoscopy reduces need for liver transplant
    d. It prevents dominant strictures
    e. It detects small duct PSC earlier

15. Which colonoscopic technique is preferred for surveillance in PSC-IBD?

    a. Standard white light with random 4-quadrant biopsies every 10 cm
    b. Chromoendoscopy with targeted biopsies
    c. CT colonography annually
    d. Capsule colonoscopy
    e. Sigmoidoscopy only

16. A 29-year-old with PSC has a normal colonoscopy with biopies and no IBD symptoms. How often should future colonoscopies be performed if the patient remains asymptomatic from IBD?

    a. Every year regardless
    b. Every 5 years
    c. Only if ALP doubles
    d. Not necessary unless symptoms arise
    e. Only after liver transplant

17. A 48-year-old man presents with obstructive jaundice and an MRCP showing long-segment intrahepatic and extrahepatic bile duct stricturing. He has no history of IBD. His alkaline phosphatase is markedly elevated, and his total bilirubin is 5.8 mg/dL. On exam, he has bilateral painless parotid swelling and a diffusely enlarged pancreas on CT. Which test would be most helpful to confirm the likely diagnosis?
    a. Liver biopsy to look for onion-skin fibrosis
    b. Serum IgG4 level
    c. Colonoscopy with biopsies
    d. ERCP brush cytology and FISH
    e. Anti-neutrophil cytoplasmic antibody (p-ANCA)

18. A serum IgG4 of 310 mg/dL (ULN = 135) in PSC warrants:
    a. Steroid trial
    b. Observation only
    c. High-dose UDCA
    d. Colonoscopy to rule out IBD
    e. Pancreaticoduodenectomy

19. A 52-year-old man with PSC is scheduled for ERCP with balloon dilation and a possible stent placement of a symptomatic dominant stricture due to recent cholangitis. Which of the following is not considered an appropriate reason for providing pre-procedural antibiotics?
    a. Recent or current acute bacterial cholangitis
    b. Manipulation of the biliary tree after bacterial colonization due to the stricture can trigger acute cholangitis
    c. Antibiotics will improve the gut microbiome and will lead to positive effects in all patients with gastrointestinal disorders
    d. There is concern that there may be incomplete proximal biliary drainage
    e. Periprocedural cholangitis can lead to negative outcomes

20. A 49-year-old woman with newly diagnosed PSC asks whether she should start ursodeoxycholic acid (UDCA). Your review of the data from clinical trials shows that a dose of 28-30 mg/kg/day of UDCA in PSC is associated with which of the following outcomes?
    a. Improved transplant-free survival and fewer dominant strictures
    b. Significant reduction in colorectal cancer risk without added toxicity
    c. Higher rates of serious adverse clinical events, including variceal bleeding and need for transplantation
    d. No measurable biochemical or clinical effect compared with placebo
    e. Cure of PSC in approximately one-third of patients

21. A PSC patient with 3 bouts of cholangitis in 6 months despite adequate ERCP therapy is classified as:
    a. Uncontrolled IBD
    b. Portal hypertensive cholangiopathy
    c. Refractory cholangitis warranting transplant consideration
    d. Dominant stricture resolution
    e. Post-ERCP syndrome

22. Which of the following is not a typical PSC mimicker to keep in mind before diagnosing a patient with PSC?

    a. HIV-associated cholangiopathy
    b. Ischemic cholangiopathy
    c. Metabolic dysfunction-associated steatohepatitis
    d. IgG4 cholangiopathy
    e. Recurrent pyogenic cholangitis

23. An EUS-guided FNA/FNB of a hilar mass in a transplant-eligible PSC patient is discouraged because:

    a. It has lower sensitivity than brushing
    b. It is a high-risk procedure
    c. It requires general anesthesia
    d. Insurance will not cover the test
    e. Transperitoneal tract seeding may exclude transplant eligibility

24. Of the choices below, which is considered a primary initial therapy for a symptomatic dominant stricture in PSC?
    a. Intraductal steroid injection
    b. Balloon dilation
    c. Radiofrequency ablation
    d. Uncovered SEMS placement across the hilum
    e. Hepaticojejunostomy

25. A MELD of 13 in a PSC patient triggers transplant evaluation under which circumstance?

    a. Presence of variceal bleeding one time
    b. Isolated elevated ALP
    c. Single episode of asymptomatic bacterobilia
    d. Elevated IgG4
    e. Recurrent episodes of cholangitis

26. For malignant distal CBD obstruction that is unresectable, the best choice to minimize reintervention is:

    a. Single 10 Fr plastic stent
    b. Multiple plastic stents in parallel
    c. SEMS
    d. Percutaneous biliary drain
    e. Nasobiliary drain

27. In perihilar malignant strictures, adequate drainage typically means:

   a. Unilateral stent crossing the confluence
   b. Drain ≥50% of functioning liver volume
   c. Drain all ducts with plastic stents
   d. Place a covered Y-metal stent across the hilum
   e. Percutaneous biliary drainage of the right system only

28. Of the choices below, which medication has the most evidence for relieving cholestatic pruritus in PSC after bile acid sequestrants fail?

   a. Acetylsalicylic acid
   b. Ursodeoxycholic acid 13 mg/kg
   c. Vancomycin
   d. Rifampin
   e. Oxycodone

29. The principal reason to avoid ERCP stent placement across the cystic duct in PSC is:

   a. It increases pancreatitis risk
   b. It can precipitate acute cholecystitis
   c. It reduces FISH sensitivity
   d. It lowers stent patency
   e. It causes immediate hemobilia

30. A 9-mm gallbladder polyp discovered on annual ultrasound in an asymptomatic PSC patient should prompt:

   a. Six-month ultrasound follow-up
   b. MRCP every 3 months
   c. Elective cholecystectomy
   d. Endoscopic polypectomy
   e. Observation until polyp reaches 15 mm

Answers to Biliary Guidelines Quiz

1.	B	16.	B
2.	D	17.	B
3.	C	18.	A
4.	E	19.	C
5.	A	20.	C
6.	B	21.	C
7.	C	22.	C
8.	A	23.	E
9.	B	24.	B
10.	C	25.	E
11.	E	26.	C
12.	B	27.	B
13.	A	28.	D
14.	B	29.	B
15.	B	30.	C

Chapter Three

LIVER ME TIMBERS!

A Voyage Through the Storms of Hepatic Disease

If the pancreas is a bag of enzymes with a temper and the biliary system is a tangle of booby-trapped plumbing, then maybe the liver is the weary captain at the helm—stoic, uncomplaining, and quietly juggling 500 jobs at once. It detoxifies, synthesizes, stores, excretes, regulates, and reboots. Most of the time, it does all of this silently. But when it decompensates, it doesn't whisper. It screams!

In this chapter, we set sail across the full arc of hepatic medicine—through quiet currents, sudden squalls, and, yes, the occasional Category 5 disaster. We begin with Alcohol-Associated Liver Disease, including all its clinical, social, and ethical complexities. Then we go to the Evaluation of Abnormal Liver Chemistries, where we ask hard questions about what's "normal," and what's not, and what subtle lab signals deserve more respect than they get.

From there we see how the liver suddenly can unravel into Acute Liver Failure and into Idiosyncratic Drug-Induced Liver Injury, a condition with no rules except one: Expect the unexpected. We follow with the intricacies of Acute on Chronic Liver Failure, yet another dramatic disease process with high mortality, limited window for intervention, and the ever-present question: Is it time to call transplant?

The chapter also covers Focal Liver Lesions, including how to sort harmless hemangiomas from dangerous hepatocellular carcinomas (HCCs) without panicking over every incidentaloma, and Liver Disease in Pregnancy, where we'll walk through the major players – from preeclampsia to HELLP to acute fatty liver and clarify when it's the pregnancy that threatens the liver, and when it's the other way around.

We'll navigate the tricky terrain of Hereditary Hemochromatosis, where iron overload masquerades as everything from diabetes to arthropathy, and then tackle the hepatic and mesenteric circulation to show how smooth currents can get suddenly blockaded and end up with a natural disaster.

So yes, this chapter is big. But it has to be. The liver sits at the center of almost everything we do in GI—and when it fails, it takes the rest of the system with it. These ACG guidelines help us recognize trouble early, manage it wisely, and know when to push for escalation.

Let's get going. There's a lot of water ahead.

Case 3.1: Diagnosed with Sinusitis

A 23-year-old woman living with obesity and a history of anxiety presents to urgent care with 3 days of sinus congestion, headache, nausea, and vomiting. She also mentions several months of persistent fatigue. When asked about alcohol use, she admits to drinking "a good amount of wine" daily to help manage her anxiety. She does not routinely see a doctor and has no known medical problems. She has not experienced jaundice, fever, abdominal pain, or edema.

On exam, she appears anxious but is otherwise well-appearing. No stigmata of chronic liver disease are noted.

Laboratory results: AST 97 IU/L; ALT 41 IU/L; alkaline phosphatase 108 IU/L; GGT 89 IU/L; total bilirubin 1.0 mg/dL; MCV 104 fL; WBC 7.1 × 10^9/L; hemoglobin 13.9 g/dL; platelets 204 × 10^9/L.

Abdominal ultrasound reveals diffuse hepatic echogenicity consistent with steatosis. The spleen and gallbladder are normal.

She is diagnosed with sinusitis and sent home with decongestants and antibiotics.

Know your guidelines!

1. What else should have been done in evaluating her abnormal liver tests?
2. How should the elevated AST, GGT, and macrocytosis be interpreted in the context of alcohol use?
3. Does this patient meet criteria for additional testing or referral for suspected ALD?
4. How might this case evolve if no intervention is made?
5. What role does GGT play in evaluating suspected alcohol-associated liver injury?

Case 3.1: What do the guidelines say?

Source: ACG 2024 Clinical Guideline: Alcohol-Associated Liver Disease[75]

Screen for alcohol use at every healthcare encounter to prevent downstream consequences

Life—and clinical practice—is full of lessons from missed opportunities. This case is one of them. A young woman presented with subtle but classic signs of alcohol-associated liver disease (ALD), and it flew under the radar. Had her alcohol use been recognized and addressed earlier, it might have altered her long-term trajectory. That's why it's essential to screen for alcohol use disorder (AUD) at every healthcare encounter—not just in liver clinic, but wherever patients show up.[76] We routinely care for patients with unrecognized AUD who present with fatigue, mental health concerns, or vague GI complaints. If we identify the pattern early and offer intervention, we can prevent the downstream consequences we all know too well.

Now, a quick but important detour—we'll call it Soapbox Time.

Use the proper terminology for alcohol-associated conditions

Language matters. We should all move away from labeling patients as "alcoholics." It's a loaded word, steeped in stigma, and often carries baggage shaped by pop culture, not medicine. Instead, we should describe conditions as "alcohol-associated"—as in alcohol-associated hepatitis, alcohol-associated liver disease, or alcohol-associated cirrhosis. These terms reflect the clinical reality without reducing a person to a behavior or diagnosis. See **Table 3.1** for more.

Table 3.1. *Updated Nomenclature for Alcohol-Associated Conditions.*

Old Term	New Term
Alcohol abuse	Alcohol misuse
Alcoholism	Alcohol use disorder (AUD)
Alcoholic	Person with AUD
Alcoholic hepatitis	Alcohol-associated hepatitis (AH)
Alcoholic liver disease	Alcohol-associated liver disease (ALD)

Why does this matter? Because stigmatizing language delays care. It pushes patients away from the healthcare system, discourages them from seeking help, and ultimately, contributes to later-stage presentation and worse outcomes. On a broader scale, stigma also impacts policy, funding, and access to treatment—when conditions are viewed as "self-inflicted," they're less likely to receive research dollars and public support.

We want to open doors, not close them. Early intervention works. Changing how we talk about alcohol-related disease is part of changing how we treat it.

Back to our patient

To screen for AUD, the Alcohol Use Disorders Identification Test (AUDIT) is a validated 10-question tool with strong sensitivity and specificity.[77] That said, it can be a bit unwieldy in busy clinical settings. For everyday practice, the AUDIT-C—a concise, 3-question version focused on alcohol use in the past year—is often more practical.

AUDIT-C is a quick 3-question tool that can be done at most health encounters to identify hazardous drinking

As shown in **Table 3.2**, the AUDIT-C has been validated across diverse patient populations and remains a reliable screening tool

Table 3.2. *AUDIT-C Questionnaire.*

Question	Scoring Points
How often do you have a drink containing alcohol?	0 = Never 1 = Monthly or less 2 = 2–4 times a month 3 = 2–3 times a week 4 = 4 or more times a week
How many drinks do you have on a typical day when you are drinking?	0 = 1 or 2 1 = 3 or 4 2 = 5 or 6 3 = 7 to 9 4 = 10 or more
How often do you have 6 or more drinks on 1 occasion?	0 = Never 1 = Less than monthly 2 = Monthly 3 = Weekly 4 = Daily or almost daily

for identifying hazardous drinking. Points are determined by the corresponding amount or frequency of drinking. Scores of 5 or more are particularly suggestive of an underlying AUD and should prompt further evaluation.

Alcohol-Associated Liver Disease: A Growing Tide

ALD is a growing global health problem, including here in the U.S. It now ranks as a leading cause of liver-related morbidity and mortality, and unfortunately, the numbers are headed in the wrong direction.[78,79] Over the past decade, the prevalence of ALD has been rising, especially among young adults, women, and historically marginalized populations like Hispanic and Native American communities.[80]

The COVID-19 pandemic didn't help matters—alcohol consumption increased by roughly 14% compared to pre-pandemic levels, and there's been no sign of that trend reversing.[81] In fact, as hepatitis C therapy revolutionized outcomes and reduced liver transplant need, ALD has quietly become the most common indication for liver transplantation in the U.S.[82]

> Alcohol misuse increased during the COVID-19 pandemic and has not decreased since

So why are we so confident this patient has ALD? Start with the pattern: an AST:ALT ratio >2, elevated GGT, and macrocytosis (MCV 104)—that's the classic biochemical fingerprint. Add her self-reported alcohol use and the absence of other causes, and the clinical picture becomes hard to ignore.

> PEth testing can distinguish moderate from heavy drinking in the past month and can be used to monitor ongoing use of alcohol

If confirmation is needed, direct alcohol biomarkers can be helpful. These include urine ethyl glucuronide, blood alcohol concentration, and—most usefully—serum phosphatidylethanol (PEth). PEth is particularly valuable because it distinguishes moderate from heavy drinking over the prior ~28 days, and can be used to monitor ongoing use.[83]

What Should We Recommend?

Now that we've recognized ALD, we have an opportunity. There are effective interventions that can change the trajectory of AUD and, by extension, liver health. Non-pharmacologic therapies include cognitive behavioral therapy, motivational enhancement therapy, and 12-step facilitation programs like Alcoholics Anonymous—all of which are evidence-based and work well.

An integrated, multidisciplinary care model works best for alcohol use disorder

Pharmacologic treatment is also important and guideline-endorsed. Medications can reduce relapse, slow disease progression, and improve outcomes in patients with cirrhosis.[84,85] **Table 3.3** outlines medication-assisted treatment (MAT) options within an integrated, multidisciplinary care model.

One option to highlight: baclofen, which has been shown to be safe and effective in patients with compensated ALD. On the other hand, disulfiram, while still FDA-approved for AUD, should be avoided in anyone with liver disease—it's metabolized entirely by the liver and carries a real risk of hepatotoxicity.

Early recognition, supportive language, and evidence-based treatment—this is how we meet ALD head-on, rather than waiting for it to declare itself in the transplant evaluation.

It's crucial to recognize that diagnosing and managing ALD requires a multidimensional approach.[87] Screening for AUD with tools like the AUDIT-C helps clinicians assess risk and identify patients who may benefit from further intervention. But the work doesn't stop there.

Medications can help with management of ALD in combination with cognitive behavioral therapy as AUD is a global disorder

Once ALD is identified, the focus shifts to comprehensive management—not just of the liver disease, but of the behavioral drivers fueling it. Cognitive behavioral therapy, motivational enhancement therapy, and similar strategies have proven effective in supporting patients with AUD. These aren't just add-ons—they're core interventions. Patients need to be referred at first presentation.

Table 3.3. *FDA-approved and Non-FDA-approved Medications for AUD.*[86]

Medication	Dosage	Pharmacologic target	Possible use for AUD in patients with ALD
FDA-approved medications for AUD			
Disulfiram	250-500 mg QD	Inhibition of aldehyde dehydrogenase	No (hepatic metabolism); cases of liver toxicity reported
Naltrexone	PO: 50 mg QD IM: 380 mg monthly	Mu opioid receptor antagonist	With caution, perceptions of liver toxicity limit use in advanced ALD
Acamprosate	666 mg TID	Possible NMDA receptor agonist	Yes (no hepatic metabolism)
Non-FDA-approved medications tested for AUD			
Balcofen	10 mg TID, 80 mg QD max	GABA-B receptor agonist	Yes (minimal hepatic metabolism)
Gabapentin	900-1,800 mg QD	Modulates GABA conduction	Yes (no hepatic metabolism)
Topiramate	300 mg QD	Anticonvulsant, multiple targets; glutamate, GABA	Yes (partial hepatic metabolism by glucuronidation); caution in hepatic encephalopathy

Because here's the truth: if you don't address why someone is drinking, you're just chasing lab values while the underlying fire keeps burning.

AUD is a global disorder that lives at the intersection of biology, psychology, and social circumstance. And until we address all 3, we're not truly treating it.

In parallel, patients with ALD need ongoing monitoring. Routine liver tests and imaging can help catch disease progression early—before decompensation sets in—and offer windows for meaningful intervention.

Bringing It Together

This case reminds us that ALD isn't a one-note diagnosis—it's a complex, dynamic condition that sits at the center of liver medicine, psychiatry, and public health. We have tools to detect it early (like AUDIT-C), biomarkers to track it (like PEth), therapies to treat it (behavioral and pharmacologic), and clinical patterns to recognize it (AST:ALT >2, macrocytosis, elevated GGT).

But above all, it takes clinical curiosity and compassion. We must meet patients where they are, offer them a path forward, and remind ourselves that the most powerful treatment we have might just be recognizing the problem before the liver fails.

Case 3.2: From Book Club to Biopsy

Ten years have passed, and our patient is now 33. Since her last visit, she's undergone gastric bypass surgery, joined a book club, and developed a fondness for wine—and the occasional espresso martini when the plot gets particularly gripping. She reports finishing 1 to 2 bottles of wine per day, which, while not in the syllabus, has become part of her reading ritual.

She presents to the ED with a week of feeling unwell, including new right upper quadrant pain, jaundice, and low-grade fevers over the past 2 days. She also notes that she quit smoking last week—perhaps because she wasn't feeling well, or perhaps in a moment of insight. Her father died young from complications of alcohol-associated liver disease, and the concern seems to be sinking in.

Vitals: T 99.5°F; BP 110/78; HR 92; BMI 30

Exam: Jaundiced, with RUQ tenderness but no guarding or peritoneal signs.

Labs: Total bilirubin 2.9 mg/dL; ALP 153 IU/L; INR 1.2; AST 231 IU/L; ALT 120 IU/L; creatinine 0.7 mg/dL; lipase 120 U/L; WBC 12.1×10^9/L; hemoglobin 13.2 g/dL; platelets 138×10^9/L; AFP 3.8 ng/mL.

Ultrasound: Hepatomegaly, cholelithiasis, no bile duct dilation, no ascites.

Initially, general surgery is consulted for possible cholecystectomy. But after reviewing the imaging and labs, they opt to pursue a liver biopsy to further evaluate the underlying liver disease. You're now consulted to interpret the pathology (see **Figure 3.1**) and weigh in on next steps.

Figure 3.1. *Liver Biopsy.*

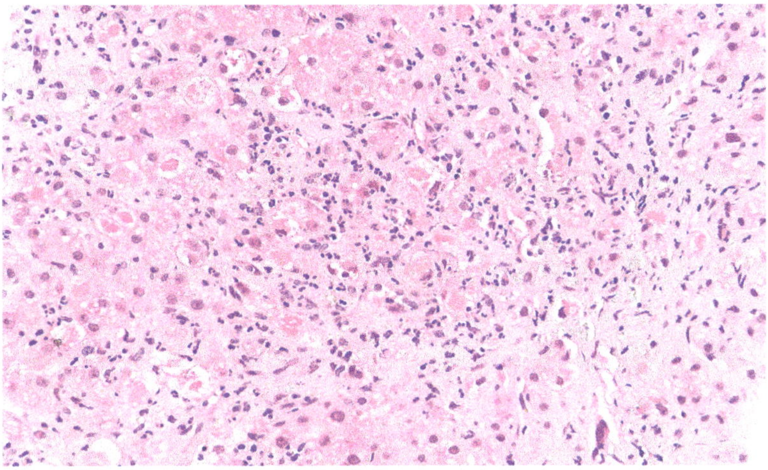

Know your guidelines!

1. What is the primary cause of her current presentation?
2. What risk factors likely contributed to her liver disease?
3. How does family history contribute to risk?
4. What nutritional strategies are important in managing her illness?

Case 3.2: What do the guidelines say?

Source: ACG Clinical Guideline: Alcohol-Associated Liver Disease[75] and ACG Malnutrition and Nutritional Recommendations in Liver Disease[88]

Well, we know this isn't cholecystitis. Even though the patient presents with Charcot's triad—fever, right upper quadrant pain, and jaundice—this isn't ascending cholangitis. It's alcohol-associated hepatitis (AH), and like many AH cases, it's easy to miss. Right upper quadrant pain can result from stretching of Glisson's capsule due to hepatic inflammation. AH often includes a low-grade fever and leukocytosis from systemic inflammation as well.

> RUQ pain in AH can result from stretching of Glisson's capsule from the hepatic inflammation

Her liver biopsy shows the classic features of alcohol-associated steatohepatitis: numerous ballooned hepatocytes with Mallory-Denk bodies, intense neutrophilic inflammatory infiltrate and perisinusoidal fibrosis. Unfortunately, the wine hasn't been kind to her liver. She has moderate AH with a MELD of 12, so at least we do not have to think about steroids at this point. Stay tuned for more about that.

Risk Factors

Let's review the risk factors—because she's got a bunch of them. First the alcohol. This is the primary culprit, no doubt. After all, this is a clear-cut case of AH given the liver biopsy findings in combination with the large amount of alcohol consumption—1 to 2 bottles of wine daily is a lot! Even more than 1 drink per day can be risky for women; more than 2 per day increases the risk in men. Binge drinking is especially harmful. Second, she's living with obesity, which independently increases the risk of liver injury in those consuming more than 3 drinks per day.[89] So, if she was drinking a smaller amount of alcohol—say 1 to 2 bottles of wine per week, then we could entertain the notion that MetALD (metabolic and alcohol-associated liver disease) is at play here. However, she is

> Obesity and alcohol misuse independently increase the risk for liver disease and HCC

not a moderate drinker. She is drinking far too much, confirmed by her liver biopsy demonstrating the acute inflammatory alcohol-related changes of straight-up AH rather than MetALD. But while we are on the topic of MetALD, you ought to know that metabolic dysfunction and alcohol work together to accelerate liver damage in MetALD. That is, alcohol misuse and obesity independently increase the risk for liver disease and appear to act synergistically even at low alcohol consumption (below 3 drinks per day).[90] It's a 1-2 punch that increases the risk not only of cirrhosis, but also HCC.[91] Unfortunately, MetALD is on the rise—thanks to increasing rates of both AUD and obesity. So be on the lookout for it in clinic.

> MetALD is on the rise—thanks to increasing rates of both AUD and obesity

What about genetics? We've all seen patients who drink heavily for decades with no liver disease—and others who develop cirrhosis with less consumption. Only 10%–20% of heavy drinkers develop cirrhosis, which tells us something genetic is at play. For example, women are more vulnerable to ALD at lower levels of alcohol consumption, likely due to lower gastric alcohol dehydrogenase activity and higher body fat composition.[92] And this patient may be genetically predisposed: individuals with the PNPLA3 rs738409 homozygous genotype are more likely to develop AH[93] and to experience worse outcomes.[94]

> Women are more vulnerable to ALD than men

> Those with PNPLA3 rs738409 homozygous genotype are more likely to develop AH and have disease progression

Her gastric bypass surgery also puts her at elevated risk. AH is 2 to 3 times more common in patients with post-bariatric anatomy.[95] Why? The reasons are likely multifactorial: a smaller stomach means less alcohol dehydrogenase enzyme, while faster transit to the small intestine allows for more rapid absorption. On top of that, some patients who previously used food to self-soothe may substitute alcohol post-surgery. All of this adds up to more liver damage. That's why screening for AUD before and after bariatric surgery is essential.

She should also be counseled about smoking cessation. Smoking

Smoking and post-bariatric anatomy are risk factors for ALD

increases hepatic fibrosis, and one large study of over 100,000 people found a threefold increase in alcohol-related cirrhosis among smokers.[96] The effect is even more pronounced in women than men.[97]

Nutrition assessment is another cornerstone of managing ALD. Guidelines specifically recommend nutrition screening in all patients with ALD—especially those with AH—due to the high prevalence of malnutrition and anorexia. In fact, malnutrition is nearly universal in severe AH.[98] So, if you're seeing a patient with AH, you should assume there's some degree of nutritional deficiency.

Malnutrition is nearly universal in severe AH

Nutritional supplementation should be part of the treatment plan for patients with AH or cirrhosis. Our patient has a BMI of 30, which is right around the average BMI in U.S. patients with ALD. But don't let the BMI fool you—many of these patients are malnourished. This is the concept of sarcopenic obesity: patients who are overweight or obese but still suffer from severe muscle loss and metabolic compromise.[99] To improve lean muscle mass and reduce the risk of complications like ascites and hepatic encephalopathy, the guidelines recommend late evening snacks in patients with cirrhosis. The goal is to promote glycogen storage and prevent overnight fasting-induced muscle breakdown. For inpatients with ALD or cirrhosis, early initiation of oral or enteral nutrition is essential. For outpatients, frequent small meals—including a bedtime snack between 7 and 10 p.m.—can help maintain muscle mass and caloric intake to prevent malnourishment. Nutritional support can make a huge difference for these patients as noted in **Figure 3.2.** In particular, those with hepatic encephalopathy, it is particularly important to encourage a plant-based protein enriched diet to maintain lean muscle mass. Moreover, stay away from high fructose containing foods, which can contribute to hepatic inflammation. Thus, a low-fructose diet is recommended for all patients with chronic liver disease.

Late evening snacks are recommended for alcohol-associated cirrhosis to prevent muscle breakdown

And while alcohol may be calorie-dense, it's nutritionally empty. It often displaces actual food and contributes to micronutrient deficiencies. **Table 3.4** outlines the common vitamin and mineral deficiencies seen in ALD, along with their clinical consequences.

Figure 3.2. *Sarcopenic Obesity With Improved Muscle Mass After Nutrition Support.*[100]

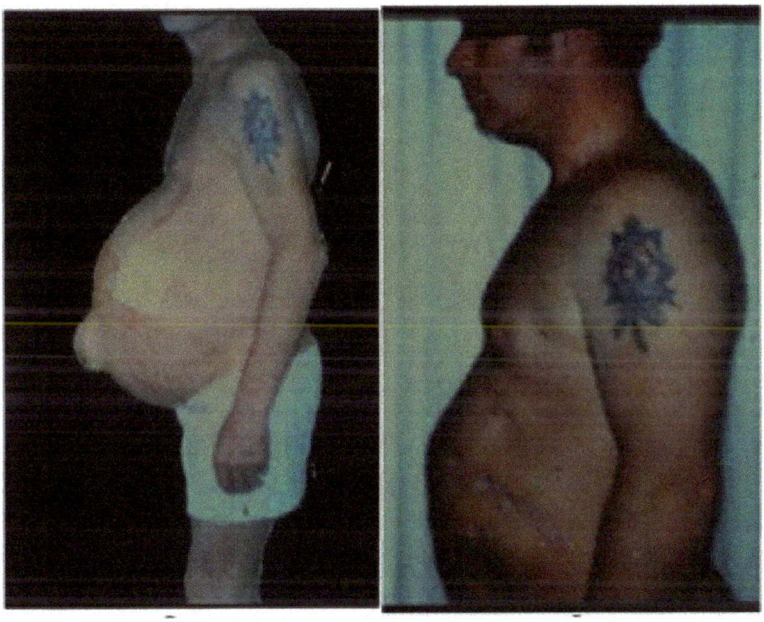

Table 3.4. *Mineral and Vitamin Deficiencies With Associated Complications in Liver Disease.*[88]

Nutrient	Signs & Symptoms
Iron	Anemia, fatigue
Magnesium	Muscle cramps, weakness, insulin resistance, low bone density
Calcium	Decreased bone density, tetany
Zinc	Anorexia, poor wound healing, diarrhea, immune dysfunction

Fortunately, she's motivated. She's stopped drinking, agreed to a referral for cognitive behavioral therapy, and has enrolled in a multidisciplinary AUD relapse prevention program with support from her primary care doctor, a mental health provider, and her GI team.

> Coffee consumption is inversely associated to fatty liver, fibrosis progression, and HCC

Since she likes coffee, go ahead and encourage her to keep drinking it—ideally 2 to 4 cups a day. Why? Because coffee isn't just a morning ritual; it's medicine for the liver. This is not new information. We even discussed the hepatological benefits of coffee consumption in our first textbook together many years ago.[101] Since then, multiple large-scale epidemiologic studies have shown that coffee consumption is inversely associated with fatty liver, fibrosis progression, and even hepatocellular carcinoma (HCC). Just be sure to clarify that this means actual coffee—not espresso martinis. Fortunately, she's vowed to stay off alcohol and has been referred to a comprehensive relapse prevention program that includes cognitive behavioral therapy, follow-up with her PCP and mental health provider, and continued care with her gastroenterologist.

Bringing It Together

This wasn't cholangitis or cholecystitis—it was alcohol-associated hepatitis, hiding in plain sight. Fever, RUQ pain, leukocytosis, and jaundice? Classic AH. And her biopsy told the rest of the story: ballooned hepatocytes, Mallory-Denk bodies, neutrophils, and fibrosis.

She checks every risk box: obesity, binge drinking, gastric bypass, possible PNPLA3 variant, and smoking. Even though alcohol is by far and away the primary culprit of her liver problems, these risk factors can drive disease progression.

Nutritionally, don't be fooled by her BMI. Sarcopenic obesity is common in AH, and malnutrition is nearly universal in severe cases. She needs late-night snacks, early nutrition, and targeted supplementation.

The bright spot? Coffee. Two to 4 cups a day (hold the martini) may help slow fibrosis and reduce HCC risk. And with a solid sobriety plan in place—including cognitive behavioral therapy and multidisciplinary follow-up—she's on the right track.

Insight, nutrition, and support: that's her path forward.

Case 3.3. Family Concerns

Five more years have passed. Our patient is now 38 years old. Unfortunately, her close friend tragically died in a motor vehicle accident recently, which prompted her to resume drinking as a coping mechanism for the associated stress. She has been drinking a handle (1.75-liter bottle) of vodka daily for the past few weeks. Her family, concerned that she "looks yellow and might be pregnant," brought her to the ED. She reports profound fatigue, dark cola-colored urine for the past week, and a sensation of abdominal fullness. She denies abdominal pain, fever, or recent sexual activity over the past 6 months.

On exam, she appears anxious but is alert without asterixis. Her skin and sclerae are icteric. She has spider angiomas, palmar erythema, and moderate ascites without tenderness. She also has bilateral lower extremity edema. Her temperature is 98.9°F, blood pressure 109/64 mmHg, heart rate 102 bpm, and BMI 28 kg/m^2.

Initial laboratory studies show total bilirubin 17.2 mg/dL, AST 190 U/L, ALT 89 U/L, ALP 201 U/L, albumin 3.0 g/dL, creatinine 0.7 mg/dL, sodium 135 mmol/L, potassium 3.5 mmol/L, and INR 2.4. Her WBC is 13.1 $\times 10^9$/L, hemoglobin 11.4 g/dL, MCV 102 fL, platelet count 64 $\times 10^9$/L, and AFP 4.1 ng/mL.

Abdominal ultrasound shows a shrunken liver without discrete masses and moderate ascites. Diagnostic paracentesis yields 3 liters of fluid, with total protein 1.2 g/dL, albumin 1.3 g/dL, total white blood cell count 56/mm^3, a negative Gram stain, and culture pending. Urinalysis is positive for urobilinogen but otherwise unremarkable. Pregnancy test is negative.

She is admitted for possible alcohol withdrawal and nutritional support.

Know your guidelines!

1. What is the next step in management?
2. If there's no improvement, is it time for hospice care?

Case 3.3. What do the guidelines say?

Source: ACG Clinical Guideline: Alcohol-Associated Liver Disease[75]

She has been appropriately admitted for close monitoring of alcohol withdrawal and should be started on oral nutrition, with enteral supplementation if she is unable to tolerate it. She also meets criteria for severe alcohol-associated hepatitis (AH), with a MELD score of 27. A MELD score greater than 20 places her in the severe AH category. By contrast, a MELD of 20 or below is considered moderate AH, where patients are generally expected to survive with abstinence and nutritional therapy. Previously, her MELD score had been lower.

Historically, the Maddrey discriminant function (MDF)[102] was commonly used to assess AH severity, with an mDF ≥ 32 associated with a 1-month mortality rate of 20%-50%.[103] However, the MELD score is now preferred, as it more accurately predicts mortality by incorporating creatinine, which is particularly helpful in forecasting outcomes in AH. The original MELD and its newer versions—MELD-Na and MELD 3.0—are considered reliable and accurate too.

> MELD score accurately predicts mortality in AH and a MELD > 20 is categorized as severe AH

Thankfully, she shows no evidence of infection or spontaneous bacterial peritonitis (SBP). Her serum ascites albumin gradient (SAAG) is greater than 1.1, consistent with portal hypertension, which can result from either severe AH and/or cirrhosis.

So, should steroids be considered? Sometimes, things in medicine don't change all that much—and corticosteroids are a perfect example. They've been studied in severe AH for more than 50 years, with dozens of trials conducted. An updated meta-analysis showed that corticosteroids reduce short-term mortality by 36%.[104] However, they do not appear to improve outcomes or survival beyond the first month. To date, no other medication has demonstrated a significant long-term mortality benefit in AH. In fact,

> Steroids improve 30-day mortality in severe AH but do not improve long-term survival

many drugs have landed in the graveyard of failed therapies, though several more are currently in clinical trials aiming to help patients with severe AH.

Pentoxifylline and prophylactic antibiotics do not help severe AH

For now, corticosteroids remain the best available option. Prednisolone is used rather than prednisone, as the latter requires hepatic conversion to the active form—something that may be impaired in severe AH. The typical dose is prednisolone 40 mg daily, tapered for 28 days.

MELD 25-39 is the "sweet spot" for steroid benefit in severe AH

Before starting steroids, it's important to ensure the patient is an appropriate candidate. The "sweet spot" for benefit appears to be a MELD score in the 25–39 range. Patients with a MELD of 40–50 derive limited benefit, and those with a MELD above 50 are unlikely to benefit at all. In addition, other medical issues must be addressed and stabilized before initiating corticosteroids, as summarized in **Table 3.5.** Targeting the right patient is essential, given the potential side effects of steroids—especially the increased risk of infection.

Table 3.5. *Contraindications for Use of Steroids in AH.*

Contraindications to steroids in AH
MELD ≤ 20
MELD > 50
Active infection (including untreated HBV)
Uncontrolled diabetes
Active gastrointestinal bleeding
Severe renal failure

After starting prednisolone, you'll want to assess treatment response early using the Lille score. While traditionally calculated at day 7, more recent data show that day 4 is just as predictive.[105] If the Lille score is ≤0.45, the patient is considered a responder, and steroids should be continued for the planned 28-day course. But if the Lille score is >0.45, that's a sign of non-response, and steroids should be discontinued to avoid unnecessary risk—namely, infection. At that point, it's time to consider alternate strategies.

Day 4 Lille score ≤ 0.45 predicts response to steroids in severe AH as well as waiting until day 7

What About Other Medications?

For a while, there was buzz around pentoxifylline, especially as salvage therapy for steroid non-responders. But the STOPAH trial[106] put that to rest—showing no mortality benefit, even in salvage situations.[107] As a result, the guideline now recommends against using pentoxifylline for severe AH. And since infection is the major downside of steroids, could prophylactic antibiotics help? Unfortunately, not really. A solid RCT showed that adding amoxicillin-clavulanate to prednisolone didn't improve outcomes compared to prednisolone alone in biopsy-proven severe AH.[108]

What About NAC?

Interestingly, N-acetylcysteine (NAC)—a star in the world of ALF—may have a supporting role here too. A network meta-analysis found that adding NAC to prednisolone in severe AH conferred a mortality benefit.[109] Based on that, the guideline recommends a 5-day course of NAC as an adjunct to steroids in patients with severe AH.

Give a 5-day course of NAC with steroids for short-term mortality benefit in severe AH

If Steroids and NAC Don't Work...

If your patient doesn't respond to prednisolone (± NAC), the best option is early referral for orthotopic liver transplantation (OLT). This should be done under strict institutional protocols, which include psychosocial evaluation, strong family support, and screening for psychiatric comorbidities that may predict relapse.

Early OLT in carefully selected patients with medically non-responsive severe AH have similar post-transplant outcomes to those with documented 6-month abstinence

Historically, patients with ALD were required to demonstrate 6 months of abstinence before being eligible for transplant. But that dogma has shifted. A pivotal French study[110] and subsequent research showed that carefully selected patients undergoing early OLT—that is, without waiting the full 6 months—fared as well or better than patients who underwent transplant after 6 months of sobriety. However, harmful alcohol use post-transplant was more common in early OLT patients, underscoring the need for ongoing AUD therapy and support even after transplant.[111]

The shift toward early OLT for medically non-responsive AH is one of the most important paradigm changes in modern hepatology—and it's reflected in the updated guidelines.

When Transplant Isn't an Option

Unfortunately, not every patient is a candidate for OLT. In cases of progressive, medically refractory AH, and when clinical trial enrollment isn't feasible, it's appropriate to involve palliative care to address goals of care, symptom management, and family support.

A visual summary of the current management approach for severe AH is provided in **Figure 3.3**.

Figure 3.3. *Management of AH.*[80]

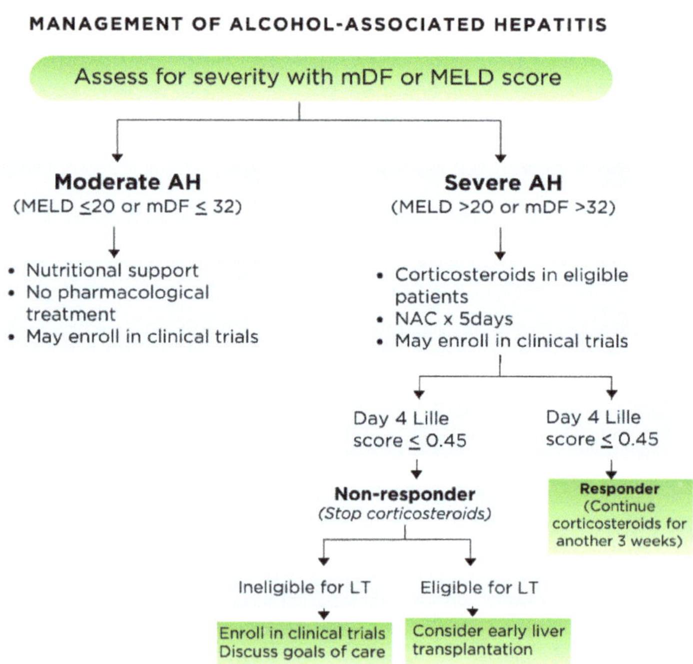

Case 3.4: A Subtle Signal

A 42-year-old man presents for an annual physical. He feels well, has no complaints, and takes no medications. His BMI is 33. Routine labs show ALT 38 IU/L (lab ULN 45), AST 30, ALP 82, total bilirubin 0.7. His primary care physician reassures him that the ALT is "normal," but you're asked to weigh in given his elevated BMI.

There's no jaundice, stigmata of chronic liver disease, or hepatosplenomegaly. No history of alcohol overuse, transfusions, tattoos, or IV drug use. Lipids show elevated triglycerides, HDL is low, and HbA1c is 6.1%.

Know your guidelines!

1. When is an ALT "normal," and when is it not?
2. What's the real ULN for ALT?
3. What's the best next step in a patient like this?
4. How does BMI influence ALT interpretation?
5. Should this patient be screened for liver disease despite having "normal" labs?

Case 3.4: What do the guidelines say?

Source: ACG 2017 Guideline on Evaluation of Abnormal Liver Chemistries[112]

This is one of the most important—and most practice-changing—messages in the entire ACG liver test guideline: a "normal" ALT isn't necessarily normal. In fact, it may be the first subtle signal that liver disease is already in play, particularly in patients with metabolic risk factors.

Rethinking the ALT Upper Limit

Many labs in the U.S. still list the ULN for ALT as 40-45 IU/L. But that number, as the guideline explains, was derived from populations that included people with obesity, undiagnosed viral hepatitis, alcohol use, and other hidden drivers of liver disease. In other words, the "normal" range was built from a not-so-normal population.

> The "real" ULN of ALT should be 33 for men and 25 for women

When you tighten the definition of health—exclude people with any of those risk factors—and look at ALT levels in truly healthy individuals, the numbers come down dramatically. The ACG guideline, echoing findings from multiple population studies, defines the real ULN for ALT as 33 IU/L for men and 25 IU/L for women.

So, our 42-year-old patient with an ALT of 38 IU/L—called "normal" by the lab—is actually above the healthy limit. That matters. Multiple cohort studies show that ALT values in this "borderline" range (35-50 IU/L) are linked to higher liver-related mortality and worse long-term outcomes.[113,114]

The Metabolic Liver Disease Link

In this vignette, the elevated ALT doesn't exist in a vacuum. The patient has a BMI of 33, low HDL, high triglycerides, and a rising A1c. This is textbook metabolic syndrome, and the leading liver manifestation is metabolic dysfunction-associated steatotic liver disease (MASLD). Yep, this was called "NAFLD" before, but let's roll with the times!

The guideline encourages clinicians to connect these dots early. In a patient like this—with metabolic risk and a confirmed ALT above the healthy threshold—MASLD is the most likely diagnosis. The goal isn't to memorize a flowchart; it's to understand the underlying reasoning and avoid premature reassurance just because the ALT slips under 40.

Here's a method of approaching modest ALT elevations such as this:

1. **Confirm**: Repeat the ALT to rule out transient elevation. ALT assays are highly reproducible—don't expect it to change much.
2. **Contextualize**: Assess for metabolic syndrome, alcohol use, and medication exposures.
3. **Investigate**: Screen for hepatitis B and C—even in patients without obvious risk.
4. **Image**: Right upper quadrant ultrasound is the test of choice for hepatic steatosis and examining the echotexture of the liver.
5. **Risk-stratify**: In those with risk factors, ultrasound-based elastography or serologic testing to assess fibrosis.

What You Don't Need (Yet)

No liver biopsy. No hepatology referral—unless your fibrosis scoring tests determine advanced fibrosis. The fibrosis 4 index (FIB-4)[115], which combines readily available laboratory values and age, is the most widely available and established tool. Moreover, FIB-4 is recommended by the American[116] and European[117] societies as a primary risk assessment tool to determine the level of fibrosis in patients with MASLD. Further follow-up and evaluation is determined by the calculated score, where FIB-4 < 1.3 is considered low-risk, FIB-4 of 1.3 to 2.67 is intermediate-risk, and FIB-4 > 2.67 is considered high-risk for advanced fibrosis. Our patient here certainly has risk factors for MASH, including elevated BMI, dyslipidemia and prediabetes, so there could be advanced fibrosis present. Nevertheless, the initial and most impactful intervention is behavioral.

Why It Matters

The reason this matters so much is because intervening early changes outcomes. A 7%-10% weight loss can normalize ALT, reduce liver fat, and even reverse fibrosis in MASH.[118] That's not theoretical. That's evidence-based, and it's actionable.

Early diagnosis of MASLD gives more time to lose weight and reverse or avoid fibrosis

If we miss the diagnosis here, we lose the chance to make that impact. By the time the patient develops more obvious lab abnormalities or symptoms, the disease is much harder to reverse.

Bringing It Together

This case captures the quiet warning signs of liver disease. An ALT of 38 IU/L may not jump off the lab report, but in the right clinical setting, it's a red flag—not a footnote.

Bottom line: Don't trust the lab's ULN for ALT. Trust the guideline. ALT values in the high 30s, especially in those with metabolic risk, should prompt a real evaluation. Early detection of MASLD gives us a window to intervene with lifestyle changes that can reverse disease before it progresses. This isn't over-calling. This is good medicine.

Case 3.5: The Curious Case of the Climbing Alk Phos

A 64-year-old woman is referred for evaluation of persistently elevated ALP. She feels well and reports no abdominal pain, itching, fatigue, jaundice, or weight loss. She takes only a multivitamin and occasional ibuprofen. She doesn't drink alcohol and has no recent travel or new medications.

Her labs, repeated over the past 3 months, consistently show: ALP 312 IU/L (ULN 120); AST 28 IU/L; ALT 32 IU/L; total bilirubin 0.8 mg/dL. Albumin, INR, and CBC are all within normal limits.

Abdominal ultrasound shows a normal liver contour, no biliary dilation, and no gallstones.

Know your guidelines!

1. How does the ACG define and approach a cholestatic pattern of liver enzyme elevation?
2. What's the role of GGT in confirming hepatic origin of ALP?
3. What's the stepwise work-up for this type of lab abnormality?
4. What are the key serologies to check?
5. What diagnoses must be considered in an asymptomatic woman with this lab profile?

Case 3.5: What do the guidelines say?

Source: ACG 2017 Guideline on Evaluation of Abnormal Liver Chemistries[112]

When AST and ALT are quietly minding their business, but ALP is climbing the walls, it's time to pivot your thinking. This is a classic cholestatic pattern of liver enzyme abnormality—and the ACG guidelines on abnormal liver chemistries give us a clean, stepwise way to tackle it. Let's go through it.

First, Confirm It's Hepatic

ALP is a notoriously nonspecific enzyme. It's made by the liver, yes—but also by bone, placenta, intestine, and kidney.[119] So, before we pin this on the liver, we need to confirm that the source is hepatic. The simplest way to do that? Add a gamma-glutamyl transferase (GGT). If GGT is elevated in parallel, it strongly suggests the ALP is coming from the liver and not from, say, osteoblastic bone activity or Paget's disease.

High ALP but normal GGT? Think bone, placenta, intestines, and kidney sources

In our patient, with normal AST, ALT, and bilirubin, but a persistently elevated ALP and a normal ultrasound, we're in prime territory to apply a focused differential. **Figure 3.4** provides a handy mnemonic to organize the causes of disproportionately elevated ALP. They spell out **LIVER MAPS**.

Think of **L**ymphoma along with other conditions that can infiltrate the liver, including sarcoidosis, amyloidosis, and tuberculosis. Next is **I**gG-4 related cholangitis, which can mimic PSC or PBC, sometimes with mass effect. Also think of **V**ascular space-filling lesions, like a large hepatic hemangioma, or a vascular hepatocellular cancer, which can compress the canaliculi and raise ALP disproportionately. **E**xtrahepatic obstruction, like from stones, strictures, or cholangiocarcinoma, might also push up the ALP disproportionately, especially if intermittent or subtle on initial imaging (over time, many of these will also drive up the transaminases and other liver tests). Reproductive etiologies of ALP might arise from the placenta, particularly during the third trimester of pregnancy when placental ALP production rises significantly. Metabolic bone disease, such as Paget's, hyperparathyroidism, or osteomalacia, can also boost ALP (but not GGT). Also think of Alcohol-associated liver disease, especially early on when ALP and GGT may rise before transaminases, although AST and ALT will eventually rise, too. PBC and sclerosing cholangitis (e.g., PSC) round out the list. See below.

Figure 3.4 *The Cause of Disproportionate ALP Elevation Spell out* ***LIVER MAPS.***

Lymphoma
IgG4-related cholangitis
Vascular lesions (e.g., hemangiomas, vascular HCC)
Extraheptic obstruction (if early or intermittent)
Reproductive / placental

Metabolic bone disease (e.g., Paget's, high PTH, osteomalacia)
Alcohol-associated liver disease (especially early on)
Primary biliary cholangitis (PBC)
Sclerosing cholangitis (PSC)

The Quiet Menace of Space-Filling Lesions

One item in this list deserves special attention: space-occupying lesions in the liver. These can raise ALP disproportionately—sometimes dramatically—by compressing canaliculi without obstructing the larger ducts. Think about how the biliary tree starts at the microscopic level. If tumor infiltration or external mass effect compresses canaliculi, bile can't flow properly, leading to cholestasis. But here's the kicker:

- AST and ALT may be normal
- Bilirubin may be normal
- Liver function may still be intact

This is what makes ALP such a subtle but powerful clue. It's a pressure indicator. When the pressure builds inside the smallest tubes first, ALP goes up long before anything else looks wrong.

That's why the guideline urges us to think about infiltrative diseases and neoplasia—even in the absence of jaundice or pain—when ALP is elevated but everything else is fine.

The Stepwise Work-Up (Straight From the ACG Playbook)

Once you've confirmed that the ALP elevation is hepatic in origin—typically through an elevated GGT, or less commonly, ALP isoenzyme fractionation—the ACG guideline lays out a stepwise approach. Start with the clinical context: consider the patient's age, sex, and symptoms. A woman in her 60s with an isolated ALP elevation? That's a textbook set-up for PBC, even in the absence of fatigue or pruritus.

Next, move to serologies. The most specific test for PBC is the antimitochondrial antibody (AMA), which, if positive, may be diagnostic without the need for further testing. An elevated IgG4 level should raise suspicion for IgG4-related cholangitis—especially if imaging shows biliary irregularities or mass effect. If there's a broader autoimmune flavor or concern for overlap syndromes, it's reasonable to check ANA and anti-smooth muscle antibody (ASMA) as well.

Woman in 60s with isolated elevated ALP →Think PBC and check an AMA

From there, imaging plays a crucial role. A normal right upper quadrant ultrasound helps exclude large duct obstruction and gallstones, but it doesn't rule out early PSC, small duct disease, or infiltrative processes. If the diagnosis remains unclear or suspicion persists, MRCP is the logical next step.

Finally, liver biopsy is not a first-line test, but it becomes important in cases where lab and imaging studies remain non-diagnostic. A biopsy can clarify infiltrative disease, confirm autoimmune hepatitis or overlap syndromes, and provide staging information when needed. In the right patient, it helps to close the loop when everything else leaves the picture incomplete.

Why This Patient? Why Now?

Our 64-year-old woman fits the classic PBC profile: middle-aged woman, asymptomatic, isolated ALP elevation. This is exactly the type of case the ACG guideline is designed to catch early. Even in the absence of symptoms, untreated PBC can progress to cirrhosis. Diagnosing it now opens the door to treatment (ursodeoxycholic acid), surveillance, and improved long-term outcomes, including decreased need for liver transplantation and a clear mortality benefit. Fortunately, the need for liver transplants due to PBC has steadily decreased, mostly attributed to early disease detection and effective treatment. For those not responding to ursodeoxycholic acid, peroxisome proliferator-activated receptor agonists show additional promise too. The future is bright for PBC patients.

Case 3.6: The Alarming ALT

A 27-year-old woman is brought to the ED at 2 AM after being found confused at home by her roommate. She has no known medical history. On arrival, she's disoriented but arousable. Her blood pressure is 106/68 mmHg, HR 98, O_2 sat 98% on room air. She is afebrile and not jaundiced. She has no stigmata of chronic liver disease, no scleral icterus, and no abdominal tenderness.

Initial labs show: ALT 3,940 IU/L; AST 4,210 IU/L; total bilirubin 1.6 mg/dL; INR 3.2; albumin 3.1 g/dL; ammonia 74 µmol/L; glucose 62 mg/dL. Creatinine is 1.3 mg/dL; lactate is 3.8 mmol/L.

A urine drug screen is pending. Her roommate reports that the patient takes acetaminophen "sometimes for migraines," has recently been stressed, and may have taken "a bunch of pills" the night before.

Know your guidelines!

1. What's the differential diagnosis for massive transaminase elevation (>15× ULN)?
2. How does the ACG distinguish between acute liver injury and acute liver failure?
3. What are the first labs you need to send in this situation?
4. When is it appropriate to refer for liver transplant evaluation?
5. What clinical and lab features predict poor prognosis?

Case 3.6: What do the guidelines say?

Source: ACG 2017 Guideline on Evaluation of Abnormal Liver Chemistries[112]

The ACG guideline draws a bright line at 15× the upper limit of normal: numbers like ALT 3,940 IU/L and AST 4,210 IU/L are a 5-alarm fire. Once you cross that threshold, you have 2 jobs, and they run in parallel: 1) identify the cause, and 2) decide—fast—whether this acute liver injury (ALI) is evolving into acute liver failure (ALF).

Transaminases >15x ULN = Five-Alarm Fire!

Step 1. Think "MAD HAVOC"

When you find AST and ALT orbiting above the stratosphere, it helps to march methodically through the handful of diagnoses truly capable of that kind of biochemical fireworks. Think "**MAD HAVOC.**"

Massive elevations most often trace back to **M**edications or toxins (acetaminophen is public enemy number one, but don't forget isoniazid, 3,4-methylenedioxymethamphetamine also known as "ecstasy," or that "natural" weight loss tea the patient might have ingested); **A**cute viral hepatitis (A, B ± D, E, occasionally a florid C, CMV, EBV, HSV); **D**emand ischemia—better known as "shock liver" after arrest, sepsis, or any profound hypotension. Then come the less obvious culprits: **H**emodynamic obstruction such as Budd-Chiari or sinusoidal obstruction syndrome; **A**utoimmune hepatitis, which can spike into the thousands when it presents fulminantly; **V**ascular toxins or infarction—cocaine, amphetamine binge, heat stroke; **O**bstetric disasters like acute fatty liver of pregnancy or HELLP; and **C**opper overload from a thunderclap presentation of Wilson disease in the young. (Severe rhabdomyolysis can imitate the pattern, so a quick CK keeps you honest.) Keep this roster in your hip pocket—Figure **3.5** lays out **MAD HAVOC** in visual form for instant recall.

Super high transaminases? Think MAD HAVOC!

Figure 3.5. *Causes of Crazy High Transaminases Spell out **MAD HAVOC**.*

Medication / toxins (e.g., acetaminophen, INH, herbals, ecstasy)
Acute viral hepatitis (A, B, $\pm$D, E, very rarely acute C)
Demand ischemia ("shock liver," cardiac arrest)

Hemodynamic obstruction (e.g., Budd-Chiari, veno-occlusive disease)
Autoimmune hepatitis
Vascular toxins / infarction (cocaine, amphetamines, heat stroke)
Obstetric catastrophes (acute fatty liver of pregnancy, HELLP)
Copper overload (rapid-onset Wilson disease in the young)

Step 2. Order the right labs now

While IV glucose drips and N-acetylcysteine are starting (NAC is beneficial in virtually every non-ischemic or non-toxic ALI scenario), send:

- **Serum acetaminophen level** (don't wait for the history)
- **Viral hepatitis panel** (HAV IgM, HBsAg, HBc IgM, HCV RNA, HEV IgM if travel, CMV IgM, EBV IgM)
- **Autoimmune markers** (ANA, ASMA, IgG)
- **Ceruloplasmin**, and if low, 24-h urine copper (or plasma-free copper)
- **Toxicology screen** (including salicylate)
- **Blood cultures & lactate** (rule out sepsis/ischemia)
- **Ultrasound with Doppler** (exclude Budd-Chiari)

Step 3. Separate acute liver injury from acute liver failure

ALT and ALF both have super high AST/ALT. But ALF also has encephalopathy

- **Acute liver injury** = huge AST/ALT $\pm$ PT prolongation, but no encephalopathy.
- **Acute liver failure** = coagulopathy (INR $\geq$ 1.5) and any degree of hepatic encephalopathy in a patient without pre-existing chronic liver disease.

Our patient already has an INR 3.2 and confusion—she meets ALF criteria right out of the gate. That automatically triggers a transplant-center phone call. The ACG guideline is clear: any ALF, regardless of etiology, deserves transfer or at least discussion with a transplant team. Timing matters; the prognosis in ALF can change by the hour.

Step 4. Understand the prognostic red flags

While King's College criteria and MELD scores quantify risk, a few findings should make you sweat immediately:

- **INR > 1.5** that keeps climbing despite vitamin K
- **Grade II or higher encephalopathy** (disorientation, asterixis, somnolence)
- **Serum creatinine rising** (hepatorenal physiology starts early)
- **pH <7.3** after fluid resuscitation (esp. in acetaminophen toxicity)
- **Factor V** < 40% in the young (or <30% in adults)

Our patient already checks 3 boxes (INR, encephalopathy, rising creatinine), so she's a high-priority transfer.

A Common Reflex—Diagnostically Dangerous

Clinicians learn early that an AST:ALT ratio > 2:1 points to alcohol-associated liver disease. True—but remember that simple alcohol-associated hepatitis by itself won't launch enzymes into the thousands. If you see AST 3,000 and ALT 1,500 and your first thought is "oh, right, that's a 2:1 alcohol-associated liver disease pattern," stop and think a little deeper. Alcohol alone never does this. Look for acetaminophen co-ingestion, ischemia from an alcohol-induced GI bleed, or a superimposed viral hit, among other possibilities.

Bringing It Together

In massive transaminase elevation, time is liver. **MAD HAVOC** keeps the differential tight, the ACG checklist keeps the work-up efficient, and early contact with a transplant center keeps options open. Even if the AST and ALT fall tomorrow (they often do as hepatic necrosis exhausts itself as the liver can run out of hepatocytes to necrose), the patient's prognosis is tied to synthetic function and mentation, not enzyme height. In fact, if the transaminases plummet, that may be a bad thing: acute liver failure may be accelerating, not getting better. So, in acute liver failure, make the call, start NAC, and let the numbers guide, but never lull you into waiting.

> A rapid drop in transaminases in ALF may be ominous. Watch the liver function tests, namely INR and TB

Case 3.7: Donor Disqualification

A 52-year-old man is referred after being disqualified from donating blood due to a mildly elevated ALT. He feels well and has no symptoms. He takes no medications, does not drink alcohol, and exercises regularly.

His labs today show: ALT 46 IU/L; AST 32 IU/L; ALP 85 IU/L; total bilirubin 0.7 mg/dL. Albumin and INR are normal. His BMI is 24, and he has no signs of liver disease on exam. He has no history of IV drug use, tattoos, or high-risk sexual exposures.

He was told by a prior provider that his labs were "fine," but the blood bank flagged him, and now he's here.

Know your guidelines!

1. How should mildly elevated ALT levels be approached in an asymptomatic patient?
2. When is it appropriate to repeat testing versus pursue a full work-up?
3. What "normal" ALT values does the ACG actually endorse?
4. Should this patient be screened for chronic viral hepatitis—even without obvious risk factors?
5. What diagnoses can hide behind the mask of "normal" liver enzymes?

Case 3.7: What do the guidelines say?

Source: ACG 2017 Guideline on Evaluation of Abnormal Liver Chemistries[112]

The very first step, before you chase zebras, is to verify that the abnormality is genuine. The ACG guideline advises a repeat chemistry panel—ideally drawn after a few days of rest, no over-the-counter analgesics, and no heroic sessions at the gym—because a brisk workout, a fistful of ibuprofen, or a simple lab mix-up can nudge ALT upward for a day or two. If that second sample slides back into the normal range, everyone gets to go home happy, and no further testing is needed. Otherwise, we'll need to dig deeper.

Redefining "Normal"

When the repeat result remains elevated, the next task is to decide what "elevated" really means. Remember from earlier in this chapter that the data-driven ULN is roughly 33 IU/L for men and 25 IU/L for women—well below the 40-plus values still printed on many lab slips. Our silent donor's ALT is 46 IU/L: only a blip by the old standard, but considerably higher than the evidence-based ULN, so it deserves a closer look.

A Stepwise Evaluation of Persistently Mild ALT Elevation

The guideline recommends a deliberate, layered evaluation that moves from common to rare without emptying the patient's wallet. Begin with metabolic and lifestyle factors: waist circumference, fasting glucose or A1c, and a lipid panel tell you whether metabolic dysfunction-associated steatotic liver disease (MASLD) is likely. A screening ultrasound (or transient elastography if your institution has it and you want to get all fancy) can confirm steatosis and fibrosis risk, and a candid alcohol history—translated into standard drinks per week—often explains a mild bump all by itself.

Regardless of reported risk factors, the next layer is universal viral screening. The CDC now calls for hepatitis C testing at least once in all adults, and our patient falls squarely into the 1945-1965

CDC says to screen for HCV in all adults born between 1945-1965 (i.e., "baby boomers")

birth cohort as well. An anti-HCV assay with reflex RNA, plus an HBsAg for hepatitis B, can catch silent infections that present only with mild transaminase elevation.

If the picture is still muddy, iron studies are in order—serum ferritin with transferrin saturation—to look for hereditary hemochromatosis; a saturation above 45% or a high ferritin justifies HFE genotyping. Autoimmune screening comes next, especially in women or those with other autoimmune hints: an ANA, an anti-smooth-muscle antibody, and a serum IgG level can unmask early autoimmune hepatitis long before cirrhosis is visible.

Selected, age-dependent tests close the net. A careful medication and supplement inventory may reveal bodybuilding pro-hormones or "detox" teas that poison the liver in silence. You can never be too careful in searching for hepatoxic ingestions. Ceruloplasmin may also be warranted to rule out Wilson disease in anyone under 40 with unexplained elevations, while a one-time α-1 antitrypsin phenotype deals with that rare deficiency if other tests have turned up empty.

A Mnemonic for the Work-Up

A handy way to keep the sequence straight is the single sentence "**ALT-TRACC**" (see **Figure 3.6** —you know much we love forcing in a mnemonic in the G2G series!). It reminds you to check: **A**lcohol and lifestyle factors, **L**ipids and metabolic markers, **T**oxins and drugs, **T**ransfusion viruses (HBV, HCV), **R**ust (iron overload), **A**uto-antibodies, **C**opper (Wilson), and **C**ongenital (α-1 antitrypsin).

Why the Work-Up Matters

Why all this effort for a number in the 40s? Because chronic hepatitis C, low-replicative hepatitis B, early hemochromatosis, and even compensated autoimmune hepatitis can hide at this level for years—and every one of them is treatable or curable if you catch it early. Conversely, a truly "normal" ALT does not confer absolute immunity; if ultrasound shows steatosis or the family tree glows with iron overload, you still address those risks directly.

Figure 3.6. *Unexpectedly High ALT? Think ALT-TRACC!*

A lcohol and lifestyle factors
L ipids and metabolic markers
T oxins and drugs

T ransfusion viruses (HBV, HCV)
R ust (iron overload)
A uto-antibodies
C opper (Wilson)
C ongenital (α-1 antitrypsin)

Bringing It Together

For our silent donor, the plan is straightforward: confirm the abnormality, then march through the ALT-TRACK sequence in an efficient, evidence-based way. More often than not, you'll uncover MASLD or mild alcohol-related elevation—both of which are reversible with lifestyle change. But if you happen to diagnose hepatitis C or hereditary hemochromatosis at this stage, you've intercepted liver disease early—when it's still fixable. That's exactly the kind of quiet win the ACG guideline is built to deliver.

Case 3.8: LFTs vs Liver Tests

A 70-year-old man is referred for evaluation of mild liver enzyme elevation. He has a history of hypertension and osteoarthritis but no known liver disease. He does not drink alcohol and is not on any anticoagulants. His primary doctor started this work-up after routine labs before cataract surgery showed: ALT 58 IU/L; AST 64 IU/L; ALP 92 IU/L; total bilirubin 0.9 mg/dL. Albumin is 3.2 g/dL and INR is 2.4.

He is asymptomatic, denies any bleeding or easy bruising, and has no jaundice, pruritus, or confusion. He takes lisinopril and acetaminophen as needed.

Know your guidelines!

1. How do transaminases relate to liver function?
2. What is the significance of an elevated INR in a patient not on anticoagulation?
3. When is albumin helpful, and when is it misleading?
4. What conditions can affect liver synthetic function without large enzyme elevation?
5. How should this patient be evaluated—and how urgently?

Case 3.8: What do the guidelines say?

Source: ACG 2017 Guideline on Evaluation of Abnormal Liver Chemistries[112]

ALT and AST tell us that hepatocytes have leaked their contents; but they do not measure how well the liver is actually working. That's why neither enzyme appears in the MELD score and why a person with acute liver failure can have normal—or even falling—transaminases while sliding into a coma. True markers of synthetic function are the proteins the liver makes (albumin; clotting factors reflected by the INR) and the compounds it clears (bilirubin). So, the next time you mention "LFTs," be sure you're referring to a real LFT and not just AST, ALT, or ALP – none of which are true LFTs. In any event, our patient's enzymes hover only one-and-a-half times the evidence-based upper limit of normal, yet his INR is 2.4 and albumin 3.2 g/dL—serious red flags that the factory, not just the smokestack, is in trouble (not sure that analogy is perfect, but we like it anyway!).

> Remember that ALT and AST are not LFTs! The true LFTs are:
> * INR
> * Bilirubin
> * Albumin

The INR Surprise

When an INR is high in a patient who is not taking warfarin or a direct oral anticoagulant, you have 3 broad possibilities: (1) genuine hepatic synthetic failure, acute or chronic; (2) factor-consumption states such as disseminated intravascular coagulation; or (3) vitamin K deficiency from malabsorption, prolonged antibiotic use, or severe malnutrition. A quick diagnostic maneuver is to give 10 mg of vitamin K: if the INR normalizes within 24 hours, the liver's synthetic machinery is intact and merely starved of cofactor. If the INR barely budges—as often happens in acute liver failure or decompensated cirrhosis—you're dealing with true hepatic dysfunction and the ACG acute-on-chronic liver failure pathways kick in (stay tuned).

> High INR? Think:
> * Hepatic dysfunction
> * Factor consumption
> * Vitamin K deficiency

Why the Enzymes Lag Behind

ALT 58 and AST 64 IU/L may look reassuringly mild, but remember

> Transaminases may start to fall—not rise—when the liver is failing. Watch liver function tests instead

2 things. First (and we can't restate this enough times), the "normal" lab slip upper limit (often 40-45 IU/L) is already inflated; modern population studies put the healthy ceiling at 33 IU/L in men. Second, as hepatic reserve dwindles, transaminase release actually falls because there are fewer viable hepatocytes left to spill their guts. You can see AST and ALT in the 50-100 range while the synthetic indices get ravaged—a classic "enzyme–function dissociation" that trips up many providers. If you've got a patient with acute liver failure, don't run a victory lap if the transaminases begin to fall. Watch the INR instead!

Building a Differential

With a high INR, low-normal bilirubin, and only modest ALT/AST, think first of broad chronic processes that erode clotting factor production without cholestasis:

- Silent cirrhosis from MASLD, alcohol, or chronic viral hepatitis
- Hereditary hemochromatosis or autoimmune hepatitis that has burned out the hepatocytes
- Unrecognized drug or supplement injury from long-term anabolic steroids or green tea extracts
- Malnutrition–vitamin K deficiency states after prolonged antibiotic courses or in the frail elderly.

Acute threats—acetaminophen toxicity, acute ischemia—usually send transaminases into the thousands and often raise bilirubin, so they are less likely here.

Next Steps—Targeted and Timely

Repeat the INR on a fresh tube, give vitamin K, and draw an expanded panel the guideline endorses: hepatitis B surface antigen and hepatitis C antibody/RNA, iron studies, ANA and ASMA with IgG level, and a good alcohol and medication history with careful attention to antibiotic and herbal supplement usage. An abdominal ultrasound with Doppler can show a nodular liver contour or portal flow changes suggestive of established cirrhosis; if it's indeterminate, ultrasound-based elastography, or MRI elastography refines staging.

Because his INR is already more than twice normal, referral to hepatology should be swift; if the INR stays above 1.5 despite vitamin K, you are in "acute-on-chronic liver failure" territory where early specialty care improves survival.

Bringing It Together

Non-GI providers often rattle off LFTs and mean AST/ALT, but the numbers that truly reflect liver function are INR, bilirubin, and albumin—the very parameters that drive prognostic scores. Our patient embodies that mismatch: modest enzymes lulled the team, but his synthetic markers shout danger. When the INR is high, believe it, and investigate fast—even if the transaminases barely blink. That's how you prevent the quiet fall from becoming a very loud disaster.

Case 3.9: NAC Time

A 23-year-old woman is brought to the ED by her roommate after being found groggy and confused in bed. She reportedly had a bad migraine the night before and may have taken "many" acetaminophen tablets, but no one is sure when or exactly how much. She has no significant medical history, takes oral contraceptives, and has no known liver disease.

On arrival, she is somnolent but arousable, with a blood pressure of 110/70 mmHg, heart rate 102 bpm, and O_2 saturation 97% on room air. She is afebrile, non-jaundiced, with no focal neurologic deficits. Her abdomen is soft and non-tender.

Initial labs show: ALT 3,640 IU/L; AST 4,020 IU/L; INR 2.1; total bilirubin 1.2 mg/dL; creatinine 1.5 mg/dL; glucose 68 mg/dL. Acetaminophen level returns at 7 mcg/mL. Serum salicylate is undetectable. Ammonia is 82 µmol/L.

She is started on IV fluids and admitted to a monitored unit. Her roommate later recalls that she may have taken the pills "sometime yesterday afternoon," but isn't sure.

Know your guidelines!

1. When should N-acetylcysteine (NAC) be started in this case?
2. What is the role of serum acetaminophen level in late-presenting patients?
3. What are the indications to extend or tailor the NAC regimen?
4. Should activated charcoal be given?
5. What other diagnoses must be considered in a young adult with massive transaminase elevation?

Case 3.9: What do the guidelines say?

Source: ACG 2023 Acute Liver Failure Guidelines[120]

The ACG guidelines treat intravenous N-acetylcysteine (NAC) as a now—not later—therapy whenever acetaminophen is even suspected in a patient with acute liver injury. The reason is pharmacokinetics: glutathione stores begin replenishing the moment NAC infuses, but the window to prevent irreversible mitochondrial injury narrows rapidly after 8 hours. By 24 hours, survival falls off a cliff if NAC has not been started. In late presenters like our patient, the rule of thumb is "treat first, clarify later."[121] You lose virtually nothing by giving NAC; you may lose a life if you wait.

Any possible chance, even a small one, of acetaminophen toxicity? Start NAC right away, and within 8 hours if at all possible!

How to Use (and Not Over-Interpret) the Serum Level

A common pitfall is to dismiss acetaminophen poisoning because the level is "low," as might be surmised in this case. But after 12-18 hours, the parent compound is already metabolized; a level of 7 µg/mL tells you only that some drug remains. The guideline reminds us that a single late level cannot rule out severe toxicity. The traditional Rumack-Matthew nomogram (see **Figure 3.7**) is only reliable when the time of ingestion is known and the level is drawn 4-24 hours afterward.[121] In unknown or staggered ingestions, your clinical clue is the combination of massive transaminase rise, early INR climb, and even a whiff of acetaminophen history.

The Rumack-Matthew nomogram is only reliable when time of ingestion is known and level is drawn 4-24 hours afterward

Dosing and When to Extend

Standard therapy is the 21-hour IV protocol (150 mg/kg over 1 h, 12.5 mg/kg/h for 4 h, then 6.25 mg/kg/h for 16 h). You should consider extending NAC if any of the following persist at hour 20:

- ALT or AST still rising
- INR > 2, or
- acetaminophen level > 10 µg/mL

Figure 3.7. *Rumack-Matthew Nomogram for Acetaminophen Toxicity.*[122]

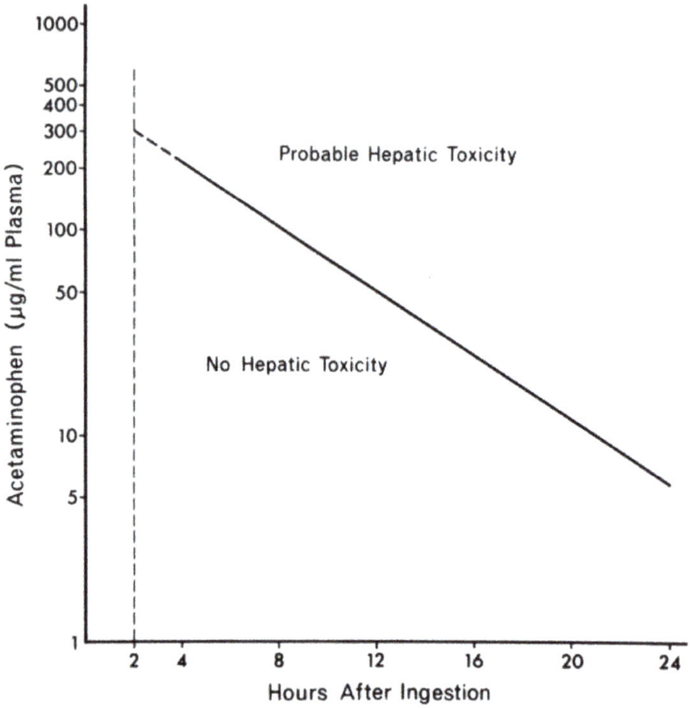

Table 3.6. *Phases and Dosing of NAC Therapy for Acute Acetaminophen Liver Toxicity.*

Phase	Rate & Duration (standard adult)	Purpose
Loading	150 mg/kg over 60min	Saturate glutathione stores
Early maintenance	12.5 mg/kg/h for 4h	Rapid detoxification
Late maintenance	6.25 mg/kg/h for 16h	Ongoing free radical scavenging
Extend	6.25 mg/kg/h for 12h	If ALT rising/INR >2/ APAP detectable

In practice, infusion continues in 12-hour blocks until ALT is falling, INR is < 2, and APAP is undetectable. **Table 3.6** summarizes NAC dosing information.

Activated Charcoal—Short Window, Big Payoff

Activated charcoal, 1 g/kg (max 50 g), still has value if it can be given within about 4 hours of ingestion, or up to 8 hours for sustained-release preparations; beyond that, gastric emptying and absorption are nearly complete.[123] In late presenters, charcoal adds little benefit, and endotracheal intubation solely to instill charcoal is discouraged.

> Use activated charcoal within 4 hours of acetaminophen ingestion

Thinking Beyond Acetaminophen

Massive aminotransferase elevation always warrants a parallel differential. Viral hepatitis panels, autoimmune serologies, Doppler ultrasound (for Budd-Chiari), and—if the alkaline phosphatase is strikingly low-serum ceruloplasmin for Wilson disease should be ordered simultaneously. But while those results incubate, NAC keeps glutathione flowing and buys time.

> Remember that if transaminases are crazy high and ALP is surprisingly low, think about Wilson disease

Prognostic Forks in the Road

With an INR already greater than 2 and a rising creatinine, our patient is rapidly approaching the threshold for **King's College Criteria (KCC)**—the most widely used tool to determine when a patient with acute liver failure should be referred for urgent transplant evaluation.[124] Developed in the 1980s and repeatedly validated, the KCC offers etiology-specific thresholds that predict extremely low rates of spontaneous survival. For acetaminophen-induced ALF, a single very low arterial pH or a triad of coagulopathy, renal dysfunction, and encephalopathy signals a need to act. For non-acetaminophen ALF, a similarly dire prognosis is suggested by either a massive INR elevation or a combination of age, etiology, bilirubin, INR, and time from jaundice to encephalopathy. The MELD score has also been found to be useful in predicting mortality for ALF.[125]

Table 3.7. *King's College Criteria for Acute Liver Failure.*[123]

Etiology	KCC for urgent transplant referral	Interpretation
Acetaminophen (APAP)	Arterial pH <7.30 (after adequate resuscitation) regardless of encephalopathy grade ***OR*** All 3: • PT > 100 s (≈INR >6.5) ***and*** serum creatinine >3.4 mg/dL (≈300 µmol/L) ***and*** • grade III-IV encephalopathy	One "pH alone" pathway, or a combined triad pathway. Fulfillment of either signals ≤20% spontaneous survival—mandating transplant evaluation.
Non-acetaminophen	PT> 100 s (INR > 6.5) regardless of encephalopathy grade ***OR*** ≥3 of the following: • Age <10 or >40 years • Etiology: non-A or non-B hepatitis, idiosyncratic drug reaction, halothane hepatitis • Jaundice-to-encephalopathy interval >7 days • PT >50 s (INR >3.5) • Serum bilirubin > 17.5 mg/dL (300 µmol/L)	Either a single very high PT or a constellation of poor prognosis factors. Meeting criteria predicts <25% transplant-free survival.

In our case, while she may not meet full criteria yet, her clinical trajectory is worrisome—and the ACG guideline is clear: transplant teams should be alerted early, not after cerebral edema or multiorgan failure has closed the window. **Table 3.7** outlines the full King's College Criteria—know them (or at least, keep them handy if you can't memorize them), and know when they apply.

Bringing It Together

Acetaminophen is still the most common cause of acute liver failure in the United States, and its antidote is cheap, safe, and time-sensitive. Start NAC immediately when acetaminophen is in the conversation—level pending, nomogram irrelevant—because delay kills. Extend the infusion while enzymes climb or INR refuses to settle, and remember that a vanishingly low drug level late in the course is no exoneration. Get the charcoal in if you're lucky enough to meet the patient early; otherwise, focus on glucose, fluids, and transplant triage. In acute liver failure, hours matter—and NAC is your first, fastest intervention.

Next case...

Case 3.10: Copper Crash

A 19-year-old woman with no known medical history presents with fatigue, nausea, and dark urine for 5 days. She reports easy bruising and mild confusion. No drug or alcohol use. On exam, she is icteric and intermittently disoriented.

Initial labs: ALT 142 IU/L; AST 168 IU/L; ALP 38 IU/L; total bilirubin 11.2 mg/dL; direct bilirubin 6.1 mg/dL; INR 3.6; albumin 2.8 g/dL; ammonia 102 µmol/L; hemoglobin 9.1 g/dL; platelets 142,000; reticulocyte count elevated. Peripheral smear shows schistocytes. Creatinine is 2.2 mg/dL. Ceruloplasmin is pending. An ophthalmology consult is requested.

Know your guidelines!

1. What lab pattern should raise suspicion for Wilson disease?
2. Why does ALP matter in Wilson ALF?
3. What is the role of Coombs-negative hemolytic anemia here?
4. How is Wilson disease confirmed in the acute setting?
5. What is the role of transplant in Wilson-related ALF?

Case 3.10: What do the guidelines say?

Source: ACG 2023 Acute Liver Failure Guidelines[120]

Wilson-related ALF is rare, but when it strikes the clock can run even faster than in acetaminophen toxicity. The ACG guidelines flag a characteristic biochemical fingerprint: modest AST/ALT elevations, a disproportionately low alkaline phosphatase (often < 40 IU/L), an ALP-to-total bilirubin ratio <4, and Coombs-negative hemolytic anemia. Our patient's ALT 142 IU/L, AST 168 IU/L, and ALP 38 IU/L in the face of bilirubin 11.2 mg/dL and INR 3.6 should set off every alarm. Unlike viral or toxic injuries—where enzymes soar—Wilson ALF produces massive hepatocellular necrosis without the enzyme fireworks, because copper's mitochondrial toxicity destroys hepatocytes so completely that few are left to leak ALT and AST.

> If the ALP:TB ratio is < 4, think about Wilson disease (especially if there is hemolytic anemia)

Oh, yeah, it's Wilson disease, not Wilson's disease. Wilson didn't have his own disease, so no apostrophe. Technically, it's also Barrett esophagus and Crohn disease, but most people throw an apostrophe on those, anyway. For some reason, Wilson consistently stays apostrophe-less. We bet you were waiting for this point to surface, so we're glad to be of service.

Why a Low ALP Is Such a Red Flag

ALP is synthesized by healthy hepatocytes and secreted into bile. In Wilson ALF, the cellular machinery is crippled, so ALP production plummets even while bilirubin climbs. A low ALP in any cholestatic picture should raise suspicion; paired with high bilirubin, it is almost pathognomonic for Wilson disease in a young patient. It's also a classic board review fact for those of you preparing for that exam.

Hemolysis: Copper's Second Attack

Free serum copper oxidizes red cell membranes, causing a sudden, sometimes fulminant, Coombs-negative hemolytic anemia. The falling hemoglobin, schistocytes on smear, and rising creatinine from hemoglobinuria all appear before the ceruloplasmin report reaches the chart. In practice, this hemolysis is often the first objective clue that something more than viral hepatitis is at play.

Confirming the Diagnosis—But Hurry to Transfer for Transplant

Low ceruloplasmin (<20 mg/dL) supports the diagnosis, yet the guidelines caution that ceruloplasmin can be low in any severe hepatic synthetic failure. More definitive tests—24-hour urinary copper >100 µg, or hepatic copper >250 µg/g dry weight on biopsy—take time the patient does not have. Slit lamp examination for Kayser-Fleischer rings is quick, and spotting them in a young adult with ALF is virtually diagnostic (**Figure 3.8**). Still, treatment decisions must precede absolute proof: if Wilson is in the differential, act fast!

Ceruloplasmin <20 supports a diagnosis of Wilson disease

Figure 3.8. *Kayser-Fleischer rings in Wilson Disease.*

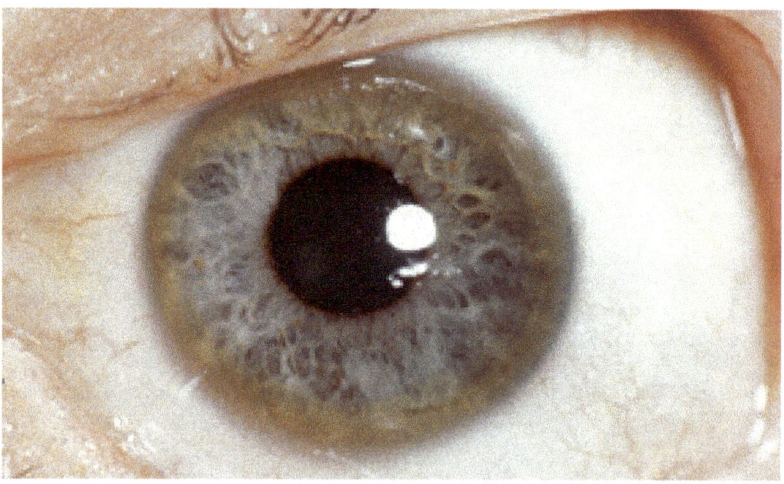

The Only Definitive Therapy Is Transplant—Early

Wilson ALF carries a mortality near 100% without a liver transplant. The guideline places these patients on the shortest leash: they should be referred for Status 1A listing at first suspicion, even before all confirmatory tests return. While arrangements are made, plasma exchange or high-flux dialysis can temporarily lower

Wilson ALF portends a nearly 100% mortality without treatment. Act fast!

serum copper, and chelators such as D-penicillamine or trientine may be started, but none are definitive. The window from encephalopathy grade II to brain-stem herniation can be measured in hours; transplant timing is everything. In fact, author HK still vividly remembers the details of this very case as a medical student where an organ did not become available in time to save this patient. A devastating and tragic outcome, which sparked his interest in hepatology.

Bringing It Together

A teenager or young adult with modest transaminase rise, very low ALP, rising bilirubin, and Coombs-negative hemolysis should scream Wilson disease until proven otherwise. Order ceruloplasmin and urinary copper, call ophthalmology for Kayser-Fleischer rings—but most importantly, call the transplant center now! We don't have a lot of time to fool around with an ophthalmoscope! (okay, nobody's "fooling around" with an ophthalmoscope, but you know what we mean). In Wilson ALF, delay is almost always fatal, and early listing saves lives.

Case 3.11: King's Move or MELD

A 46-year-old man with no known liver disease presents with jaundice, confusion, and fatigue for 5 days. He reports that he started a new herbal supplement for joint pain about 2 weeks ago (uh oh...) but denies alcohol use or acetaminophen ingestion.

Vitals: T 98.6°F, BP 104/66 mmHg, HR 96 bpm, SpO_2 96% on room air. On exam, he is disoriented to time and place, has asterixis, and is jaundiced but not in distress.

Labs: ALT 622 IU/L; AST 505 IU/L; ALP 140 IU/L; total bilirubin 21.2 mg/dL; INR 4.1; albumin 2.6 g/dL; sodium 134 mg/dL; creatinine 2.1 mg/dL; Hepatitis panel and autoimmune serologies are pending. No prior labs available. He is admitted to the ICU and NAC is started empirically.

Know your guidelines!

1. How do you distinguish ALF from decompensated cirrhosis?
2. What is the role of King's College Criteria versus MELD in transplant evaluation?
3. What are the transplant listing pathways for ALF?
4. What diagnoses should be considered in drug-induced liver injury (DILI)-related ALF?
5. How quickly should transplant evaluation be initiated in this scenario?

Case 3.11: What do the guidelines say?

Source: ACG 2023 Acute Liver Failure Guidelines[120]

The first diagnostic fork is to decide whether you are staring at a new hepatic collapse or a chronic liver that has finally tipped over. True ALF is defined by: (1) no pre-existing liver disease, (2) coagulopathy with INR ≥1.5, and (3) any degree of hepatic encephalopathy developing inside 26 weeks of a first recognized liver insult. Ultrasound shows a smooth contour, and the patient has no stigmata of portal hypertension or prior decompensation in the record. Our 46-year-old therefore fits the ALF definition on the nose: INR 4.1, grade II encephalopathy, and no past liver history.

ALF is marked by:
* No pre-existing liver disease
* INR> 1.5
* Hepatic encephalopathy

Scoring Prognosis—Why We Need Two Lenses

Once ALF is confirmed, the question is how long do we have? It's worthwhile running both KCC and MELD because each captures risk slightly differently, as outlined in **Table 3.8**.[125]

Check both KCC and MELD in ALF. They provide complementary info (see Table 3.8)

In our patient—non-acetaminophen etiology—KCC demands either a single INR >6.5 or an ominous cluster (bilirubin > 17.5 mg/dL plus INR >3.5, age < 10 or > 40, interval >7 days from jaundice to encephalopathy, or DILI/halothane etiology). He already meets 2 elements: bilirubin 21 mg/dL and INR 4.1; add the likely idiosyncratic DILI trigger, and he satisfies the "3-factor" rule—placing him below a 25% chance of spontaneous survival. His MELD 3.0 score is 42, reinforcing the gravity of the situation but offering no rescue. Together these numbers make the transplant conversation mandatory, not optional.

Status 1A: The Fast-Track Lane

For adult ALF, United Network for Organ Sharing (UNOS) grants Status 1A listing—essentially the top of the national waiting list—if patients are admitted to the ICU and certified by a qualified

Table 3.8. *King's College Criteria vs. MELD for ALF.*

Tool	Design	Pros	Cons
King's College Criteria	Rapid triage in ALF (APAP vs non-APAP paths)	High specificity. If criteria met, transplant-free survival <20%	Modest sensitivity. Some patients who die never meet KCC thresholds
MELD	Global severity, originally chronic liver disease	Continuously scaled, updated with MELD 3.0, easy to track daily and trend	Less validated in ALF. Tends to lag in early fulminant cases.

physician to have an estimated life expectancy of less than seven days without a transplant. Our patient qualifies today. The guideline urges centers to call the transplant team as soon as KCC or equivalent red flags emerge, not when intracranial pressure is already climbing.

Pinning Down the Etiology: Herbal DILI and Its Mimics

Idiosyncratic DILI accounts for roughly 10% of ALF cases in North America, and "natural" supplements—green-tea extracts, kava, bodybuilding mixes—are prominent offenders. NAC is also prudent for non-acetaminophen ALF since it has been shown to improve overall survival.[126] Don't forget that the broader work-up proceeds in parallel: viral serologies (A through E), autoimmune markers, Wilson labs in the young (especially if ALP is low), and a careful toxicology screen. If no other culprit emerges and the timeline matches, the herb becomes the prime suspect—even though confirmatory testing rarely exists.

> NAC therapy improves survival for both acetaminophen and non-acetaminophen ALF

Acting on the Scores, Not the Calendar

Time is the enemy. Cerebral edema, renal failure, and infection can close the transplant window within 24-48 hours. The ACG guideline's message is unambiguous: if a patient meets KCC or has a MELD >25 and rising, initiate status 1A listing and transfer (or activate) immediately. Waiting for "definitive etiology" or "one more set of labs" costs precious hepatocyte mass and, often, the patient's life.

Bottom line: KCC gives a clear yes/no for emergency listing, while MELD provides a dynamic trajectory; together they guide when to pull the transplant trigger. In non-acetaminophen ALF, don't let a relatively modest transaminase spike fool you—the combination of sky-high bilirubin and INR tells the real story, and the story ends badly without swift referral for transplantation.

Case 3.12: Coagulation Mirage

A 34-year-old woman with acute liver failure from presumed idiosyncratic drug-induced injury (diagnosed 2 days ago) is in the ICU awaiting transfer to a transplant center. She remains hemodynamically stable, deeply jaundiced, and intermittently disoriented (grade II encephalopathy). Overnight she develops oliguria with rising serum creatinine and is scheduled for placement of a tunneled hemodialysis catheter later this morning.

Morning labs: INR 4.5; platelets 178 × 10^9/L; fibrinogen 240 mg/dL; ALT 210 IU/L; AST 260 IU/L; total bilirubin 18.4 mg/dL; hemoglobin 11.2 g/dL. She is not actively bleeding, and her blood pressure remains 112/68 mmHg on minimal fluids. The surgical resident calls, asking, "Should we give 2 units of FFP before the line?"

Know your guidelines!

1. Why does the ACG guideline discourage routine plasma or PCC correction of an elevated INR in ALF?
2. How reliable is INR as a bleeding risk predictor in ALF?
3. Which invasive procedures, if any, warrant proactive correction—and what INR/platelet thresholds apply?
4. How should coagulopathy be managed if the patient actually bleeds during or after catheter placement?

Case 3.12: What do the guidelines say?

Source: ACG 2023 Acute Liver Failure Guidelines[120]

A prolonged INR in acute liver failure has long provoked knee-jerk plasma transfusions, yet the ACG guideline reminds us that INR measures only one side of the coagulation balance: the vitamin K-dependent pro-coagulant factors. It ignores the simultaneous fall in natural anticoagulants (protein C, protein S, antithrombin) that occurs at almost the same pace. What looks like "coagulopathic blood" in the laboratory often behaves like normally clottable blood at the bedside. There has been ample evidence showing that there is no correlation between baseline INR and procedure-related bleeding in ALF—patients bleed when they have portal hypertension with thrombocytopenia or when a vessel is nicked, not simply because the number on the chart is high.[127]

Rebalanced, Not Broken

The guideline frames ALF as a state of rebalanced hemostasis. Primary hemostasis (platelet plug formation) is frequently preserved; fibrinogen remains adequate until very late; and endothelial-derived factors tilt the scale toward normal thrombin generation despite a prolonged prothrombin time. Correcting the INR with fresh frozen plasma (FFP) or 4-factor PCC before every central line defeats that balance, adds volume (risking cerebral edema), and can blur transplant eligibility by artificially lowering INR.

When to Correct—and When to Skip It

Routine correction is not recommended for low-risk bedside procedures such as ultrasound-guided central venous access, arterial lines, paracentesis, or even lumbar puncture if platelets exceed 50 $\times 10^9$/L and fibrinogen is >100 mg/dL. Prophylactic products are reserved for high bleed risk interventions—placement of an intracranial pressure (ICP) monitor, liver biopsy, or emergency surgery—where the catastrophic consequences of bleeding outweigh transfusion downsides.

Viscoelastic Testing: A Better Compass

Remember that INR only reflects the status of vitamin K-dependent factors, not protein C, or protein S, or antithrombin

Thromboelastography (TEG) or rotational thromboelastometry (ROTEM) captures the global clotting picture—initiation, propagation, and fibrinolysis—within minutes. Some liver centers use viscoelastic testing to decide whether FFP, cryoprecipitate, or platelets are truly needed before an invasive procedure.[128] An apparently "unclottable" INR of 4 can reveal near-normal clot amplitude on TEG, arguing against transfusion. However, this is not available at most places and certainly is not the current standard of care.

If Bleeding Happens Anyway

Active hemorrhage changes the equation. In that event, the guideline endorses goal-directed therapy: PCC or FFP dosed to normalize INR rapidly, cryoprecipitate for fibrinogen < 100 mg/dL, and platelets to a threshold of 50×10^9/L. Recombinant factor VIIa is a rescue option, but only when conventional products fail and surgical control is impossible.

Bringing It Together

Remember that primary hemostasis is usually preserved in ALF until very late

Our patient's INR of 4.5 is alarming on paper, but with stable platelets, decent fibrinogen, and an image-guided dialysis catheter planned, prophylactic plasma offers more harm than benefit. The ALF guideline urges restraint: treat the patient, not the INR, consider using viscoelastic tests when available, and reserve correction for truly high-risk procedures or active bleeding. Less plasma means less volume overload, fewer transfusion reactions, and a clearer picture for the transplant team deciding her fate.

Case 3.13: Clear Skin, Cloudy Labs

A 23-year-old woman presents with fatigue and mild right upper quadrant discomfort. She has no history of liver disease, does not drink alcohol, and takes no medications—except for minocycline, which she's been using for the past year to manage cystic acne. She reports no recent travel, drug use, or illness.

On exam, she is a febrile and anicteric. There is no hepatosplenomegaly, no rash, and no stigmata of chronic liver disease.

Laboratory tests show: ALT 1,242 IU/L; AST 980 IU/L; alkaline phosphatase 118 IU/L; total bilirubin 1.4 mg/dL; INR 1.1; albumin 4.2 g/dL. Hepatitis A, B, and C serologies are negative. Her ANA returns positive at 1:160 with a smooth muscle antibody titer of 1:40. IgG is mildly elevated.

An abdominal ultrasound is unremarkable. She is referred to hepatology for concern about possible autoimmune hepatitis (AIH).

Know your guidelines!

What is the significance of this patient's pattern of liver injury?

1. How do you differentiate autoimmune hepatitis from autoimmune-like DILI?
2. Should you start steroids?
3. Is a liver biopsy indicated?

Case 3.13: What do the guidelines say?

Source: ACG 2021 Guideline on Drug-Induced Liver Injury[129]

DILI is one of the most challenging diagnoses in hepatology—not because it's rare, but because it's sneaky and dangerous. DILI is a big dilly, so you just gotta know this stuff. We've got you covered!

DILI is the most common cause of ALF

DILI can look like anything: viral hepatitis, cholestasis, autoimmune hepatitis, even early cirrhosis. But unlike those other entities, DILI is a diagnosis of exclusion, and missing it can lead to unnecessary testing, prolonged immunosuppression, or even a failure to recognize a drug you could have simply stopped. It's also not that rare: DILI is the most common cause of acute liver failure in the U.S. (with acetaminophen-induced DILI leading the list), and increasingly, it's showing up in outpatient labs, routine check-ups, and supplement-fueled mystery cases.

The ACG guideline on DILI is a much-needed roadmap. It gives clinicians a clear structure to work through the patterns of injury, triggers to recognize, and stepwise work-ups to rule out mimics. That's why in this part of the chapter, we're digging deep into the classic patterns of DILI—and this case is a perfect place to start.

Hepatocellular Injury with Autoimmune Features

This patient presents with markedly elevated ALT and AST, only a mild elevation in ALP, and a bilirubin that's modestly increased. The key to interpreting this profile is calculating the R-value, which helps categorize the pattern of liver injury. The R-value is defined as:

$$\textbf{(ALT} \div \textbf{ALT ULN)} \div \textbf{(ALP} \div \textbf{ALP ULN)}$$

Let's just assume your lab's ULN is 40 IU/L for ALT (despite earlier vignettes indicting this is probably too high) and ULN is 120 IU/L for ALP. So, if her ALT is 1,242 and ALP is 118, the R-value would be:

$$(1{,}242 \div 40) \div (118 \div 120) = 31.05 \div 0.98 \approx 31.7$$

An R-value greater than 5 is classified as hepatocellular injury, while an R-value less than 2 suggests cholestatic injury. Values between 2 and 5 fall into the mixed pattern. This simple calculation is the first—and essential—step in a suspected DILI work-up because it shapes your differential diagnosis, guides further testing, and helps determine prognosis. In this case, the pattern clearly points toward hepatocellular injury, which fits with the known profile of minocycline-induced liver damage.

> R>5 = Hepatocelluar
> R<2 = Cholestatic
> R 2-5 = Mixed

But there's more: she has a positive ANA, a positive smooth muscle antibody, and elevated IgG. This lab constellation mimics autoimmune hepatitis (AIH), and the presentation—fatigue, mild abdominal pain, no jaundice—is consistent with that diagnosis. But the key clue here is her medication history: she's been on minocycline for over 6 months, and minocycline is a textbook agent associated with autoimmune-like DILI, particularly in young women.

> Minocycline can cause an auto-immune-like DILI pattern

DILI vs Autoimmune Hepatitis—Why the Distinction Matters

Autoimmune-like DILI can be hard to distinguish from true AIH. Both can present with high transaminases, positive autoantibodies, and elevated IgG. But there are subtle differences, and the guideline urges clinicians to resist reflexively labeling these patients as "AIH" without a full evaluation.

Here's how the distinction is usually made:

- **Latency matters**: Minocycline-induced DILI typically appears after 6+ months of use.
- **Recovery is key**: After stopping the offending drug, liver tests in DILI tend to improve rapidly—often by 50% within 30 days.
- **Histology can help**: A liver biopsy may show plasma cell-rich interface hepatitis, but fibrosis is often absent in DILI, whereas AIH often shows established portal and bridging fibrosis.

In some cases, it may take time and observation to sort this out. For example, if the ALT doesn't fall by at least 50% within 30-60 days of stopping the drug, a liver biopsy should be considered, as per the guideline.

To Steroid or Not to Steroid?

AIH can show portal and bridging fibrosis on biopsy, whereas minocycline shouldn't

The ACG guideline is cautious here. Steroids should not be used reflexively just because autoimmune markers are present. In most cases of autoimmune-like DILI, the injury resolves on its own with drug withdrawal. The guideline suggests considering corticosteroids only when:

- There is diagnostic uncertainty and a biopsy cannot be readily obtained;
- The liver injury is severe or rapidly worsening;
- A true autoimmune hepatitis cannot be excluded and the patient is deteriorating.

So, in our patient's case—stable, early-stage presentation, no encephalopathy or coagulopathy—the right call is supportive care and close monitoring, not steroids.

What Next? Monitoring and Follow-Up

Once the drug is stopped, the patient should have serial monitoring of liver biochemistries every 1-2 weeks or so depending upon the clinical scenario. If ALT and AST drop by half within 30 days, and she remains asymptomatic, no further action may be needed beyond continued follow-up. The guideline emphasizes that persistent ALT elevation beyond 60 days or new symptoms like pruritus or jaundice should prompt further work-up—possibly biopsy—to rule out chronic DILI or unmasked autoimmune disease.

Crucially, rechallenge with minocycline is contraindicated. And frankly, with the availability of other, highly effective therapies for acne, it wouldn't make sense to go back to minocycline after such a serious adverse event. Moreover, recurrence can be more severe and may lead to chronic liver damage or ALF. So, that's a no-brainer.

Bringing It Together

> Autoimmune DILI culprits:
> * Minocycline
> * Nitrofurantoin
> * Methyldopa
> * Hydralazine
> * Anti-TNF

This is a classic case of autoimmune-mimicking hepatocellular DILI, and minocycline is one of the usual suspects, among a few other classics (e.g., nitrofurantoin, methyldopa, hydralazine, and rarely, anti-TNF biologics). The presence of positive ANA and smooth muscle antibody doesn't necessarily mean autoimmune hepatitis—and jumping to steroids too early can confuse the picture and expose the patient to unnecessary risk. The ACG guidelines walk us through a disciplined, structured approach: categorize the pattern, stop the offending agent, rule out other causes, and observe. And in many cases, as here, the liver just needs time—and space—to heal.

Case 3.13: Scratch that Script

A 62-year-old man presents with jaundice and pruritus 2 weeks after completing a 10-day course of amoxicillin-clavulanate for sinusitis. He reports dark urine, pale stools, and generalized itching, but no abdominal pain or fevers. He has no known liver disease and takes no other medications aside from a daily multivitamin.

On exam, he is deeply jaundiced with scleral icterus but is afebrile and hemodynamically stable. He has mild right upper quadrant tenderness without guarding or hepatomegaly.

Labs show: ALT 158 IU/L; AST 132 IU/L; ALP 426 IU/L; total bilirubin 9.8 mg/dL (direct 7.1); INR 1.0; albumin 4.1 g/dL. Hepatitis A, B, and C serologies are negative. AMA is negative. GGT is elevated. Abdominal ultrasound shows normal liver echotexture and biliary tree, with no gallstones or ductal dilation.

Know your guidelines!

1. What type of injury pattern is most typical for amoxicillin-clavulanate?
2. How should this patient be evaluated to rule out other causes of cholestasis?
3. What is the expected course of this condition?
4. What lab features define "Hy's Law," and does it apply here?

Case 3.13: What do the guidelines say?

Source: ACG 2021 Guideline on Drug-Induced Liver Injury[129]

Amoxicillin-clavulanate is the most frequently implicated prescription drug in idiosyncratic DILI throughout North America and Europe. Clinicians reach for it reflexively because it covers "everything," yet the guideline reminds us that this very ubiquity makes its delayed cholestatic injury pattern something we must recognize cold. The typical latency is deceptive: patients finish the antibiotic feeling fine, only to develop jaundice, dark urine, and relentless pruritus 1-6 weeks later—timing that often obscures the connection unless you specifically ask, "What did you take last month?"

> Amoxicillin-clavulanate is the #1 cause of idiosyncratic DILI

Pinning Down the Pattern

The first interpretive move in any suspected DILI is to classify the biochemical profile. Be sure to check the R-value, which we covered in the last vignette—the ratio of normalized ALT to normalized ALP—as your compass. In this patient ALT is 158 IU/L (ULN ≈ 40) and ALP 426 IU/L (ULN ≈ 120). Dividing each by its ULN and then dividing the 2 results yields an R just over 1, well below the cut-off point of 2 that marks a cholestatic pattern. That single calculation tells us we are dealing with bile duct-focused injury rather than hepatocyte injury, and it immediately narrows the differential to a cholestatic condition: biliary obstruction, PBC, PSC, infiltrative disease, and a short list of drugs led by amox-clav.

> Remember that R<2 means cholestatic pattern of DILI. Think of:
> * Biliary obstruction
> * PBC
> * PSC
> * Infiltrative disease
> * Amox/clav

Ruling Out the Mimics

Guideline algorithms for cholestatic DILI begin with imaging, typically a RUQ ultrasound. A normal gallbladder, nondilated ducts, and absence of mass lesion—exactly what we see here—exclude common duct stones, biliary obstruction due to neoplasm, and strictures. A markedly elevated GGT, performed in tandem, confirms that the ALP surge is hepatic rather than bony in origin. Once mechanical obstruction drops off the list, the only serology every patient truly needs is an antimitochondrial antibody to rule out unsuspected PBC; other panels (ANA, ASMA, IgG4) can be added when the presentation is atypical or imaging equivocal. But keep in mind that PBC doesn't cause the acute onset of jaundice. In classic amox-clav injury with clean imaging, further invasive studies (MRCP, ERCP, liver biopsy) are unnecessary unless bilirubin or INR keep climbing unexpectedly.

Managing the Downstream Course

There is one—and only one—disease-modifying step: **Stop the drug and never restart it.** No corticosteroid or acetylcysteine protocol hastens recovery in this setting. Skin emollients are used to help with any associated pruritus. If the itching is not improved, then antihistamines can be utilized and stepped up to other agents if needed. In general, as the liver tests decrease with time, so does the pruritus for most patients. Laboratory follow-up every 2-4 weeks reassures both patient and provider that bilirubin and ALP are trending down—although 3-6 months is a typical convalescence time frame for cholestatic DILI, which tends to resolve much slower than hepatocellular DILI. Rare patients, particularly the elderly, may plateau with a chronic vanishing duct syndrome; any failure of ALP to fall 50% by 6 months merits hepatology review.

> It can take 3-6 months to fully recover from amox-clav cholestatic DILI

Why Hy's Law Doesn't Scare Us Here

To understand why this patient isn't in danger, it helps to understand Hy's Law, a clinical principle with real teeth behind it. It's named after the one and only Dr. Hyman Zimmerman, a legendary researcher, who spent decades cataloging DILIs long before we had fancy serologies or structured reporting systems. His insight was simple but profound: if a drug causes hepatocellular injury—meaning a true rise in transaminases, not just cholestasis—and if that injury is accompanied by jaundice, the patient has about a 10% risk of dying or needing a transplant,

> Hy's Law: DILI with hepatocelluar injury + jaundice = bad.
> Look for:
> * ALT>3x ULN
> * TB>2x ULN
> * No obstruction

even if they're previously healthy.[130] That observation has since been confirmed in cohort after cohort and has become a core part of how drug safety is evaluated, including in FDA protocols and clinical trials.

To apply it correctly, 3 conditions must be met:

1. **ALT > 3× ULN**, i.e., hepatocellular pattern
2. **Total bilirubin > 2× ULN**, usually around 2.5 mg/dL or more
3. **No biliary obstruction** (i.e., clean imaging)

When those boxes are checked and no other cause for liver injury is found, the concern is that so many hepatocytes have been injured that the liver may not recover, and mortality rises. But—and this is critical—**Hy's Law applies only to hepatocellular DILI**, not to cholestatic injury like we see with amox-clav. This patient's R-value is close to 1, which makes Hy's Law not applicable, even though his bilirubin is impressively high.

In cholestatic DILI, the injury is centered on the bile ducts and canaliculi, not the hepatocytes themselves. As a result, the liver's synthetic capacity is preserved, INR stays stable, and mortality is very low—usually under 1%. That said, if bilirubin climbs above 20 mg/dL, or if INR starts creeping upward, that's your cue to reassess and possibly refer. But in the classic amox-clav case, it's discomfort and patience that dominate the course—not danger. So, thank Hy for the rule—but know when not to apply it. In this case, we can safely let the liver take its time.

In general, cholestatic DILI is less severe than hepatocellular

Bringing It Together

Amoxicillin-clavulanate DILI teaches 2 durable lessons. First, latency matters: ask about antibiotics taken in the past month, not just the past week or day. Second, pattern matters: calculating an R-value turns a sea of abnormal labs into a navigable map, directing work-up, prognosis, and follow-up. Nearly every patient recovers completely, but only if we connect the dots and "scratch that script" from their future medication list (and, in the process, prevent more scratching…). In the end, the most prescribed antibiotic is also the most predictable cholestatic culprit—forewarned, we can keep the itch, the jaundice, and the anxiety to a minimum while nature does the slow work of healing.

Next, let's keep this DILI train rolling…

Case 3.14: Checkmate

A 55-year-old woman with metastatic melanoma on nivolumab presents for routine labs prior to her fourth cycle of treatment. She feels well and reports no new symptoms. Her prior 3 cycles were tolerated without issue.

Today's labs show: ALT 396 IU/L; AST 408 IU/L; ALP 186 IU/L; total bilirubin 1.1 mg/dL; INR 1.0. She is asymptomatic and afebrile. She is not taking any new medications or supplements. Viral hepatitis panel is negative. ANA is positive at 1:80, but ASMA and IgG are normal.

She is referred to hepatology for concern about drug-induced liver injury.

Know your guidelines!

1. What liver injury pattern is typical of immune checkpoint inhibitor (ICI)-related DILI?
2. How should this case be managed?
3. Should steroids be used?
4. Need a liver biopsy?
5. Can immunotherapy be safely restarted—and if so, when?

Case 3.14: What do the guidelines say?

Source: ACG 2021 Guideline on Drug-Induced Liver Injury[129]

Immune checkpoint inhibitors (ICIs) like nivolumab, pembrolizumab, and ipilimumab have transformed cancer care—and in the process, introduced a new form of liver injury that every gastroenterologist and hepatologist now needs to recognize. As more patients receive ICIs for melanoma, lung cancer, renal cell carcinoma, and even GI malignancies, immune-related hepatotoxicity has gone from rare curiosity to regular consult. So, it's important to have a framework for diagnosis, monitoring and managementof this new DILI.

Recognizing the Pattern: Hepatocellular and Sometimes Sudden

ICI-related DILI is marked by R>5

ICI-related DILI usually presents as a hepatocellular pattern—markedly elevated ALT and AST, often >5× or even 20 × ULN, with minimal or no bilirubin elevation. So, we have a hepatocellular injury pattern here: ALT 396 IU/L, AST 408 IU/L, normal INR, and a bilirubin just above 1 mg/dL. The R-value in this setting would easily exceed 5, confirming the hepatocellular nature of the injury.

ICI-related DILI usually occurs after 3-5 infusions, not typically after the first or second

Latency varies but often occurs at 4-12 weeks or after 1-3 doses of ICIs, just as this patient is now experiencing. Unlike classic DILI, which is often idiosyncratic, ICI liver injury is immune-mediated and more predictable in timing—closer in biology to autoimmune hepatitis than to a drug reaction. That also means the injury may worsen even after the drug is stopped, due to a durable T-cell response. Low titers of ANA without ASMA are commonly found as well.[131]

The Role of Observation vs Intervention

The patient is asymptomatic, labs are quite elevated but there is no coagulopathy or encephalopathy. Nonetheless, this is categorized as a Grade 3 hepatotoxicity (ALT >5-20× ULN), which is severe, but not life-threatening (at least not yet). Obviously, the ICI needs to be at least temporarily held, and the patient should be closely monitored. Many of these cases will improve spontaneously with drug cessation. In our patient, careful observation with lab checks every few days may suffice – if the ALT continues to climb, or if bilirubin or INR increase, that's when to escalate.

When to Use Steroids—and How

While holding the ICI, if ALT or AST rise further or go beyond 20x or TB >3x ULN into the grade 4 (life-threatening) DILI or if symptoms develop (fatigue, RUQ pain, jaundice), then corticosteroids are appropriate. Either oral prednisone at 0.5-1/mg/kg/day or intravenous methylprednisolone at 1 mg/kg/day with slow tapering would be appropriate depending upon the clinical severity of hepatotoxicity. The majority of ICI-DILI cases resolve in 5-9 weeks, but deaths have been reported.

Use steroids if ALT >20x and TB >3x ULN or worsening status

Liver Biopsy: Useful but Not Always Necessary

Biopsy is not required in all cases, but it can be valuable when:

- The diagnosis is unclear
- Autoimmune hepatitis is strongly suspected
- There's a poor response to steroids
- There's consideration of rechallenging the patient with immunotherapy.

Typical histology often displays acute hepatitis with lobular inflammation and acidophil bodies (eosinophilic globules formed by dying hepatocytes) and progression to centrilobular necrosis (see **Figure 3.10**).[131] But biopsy mainly helps when management depends on knowing what's going on histologically—not when the clinical picture is already clear and improving.

Liver biopsy in ICI DILI can show acute lobular hepatitis with acidophil bodies with centrilobular necrosis.

Figure 3.10. *Liver Biopsy of ICI-Induced Hepatotoxicity. (A) Acute hepatitis with lobular inflammation and acidophil bodies (arrows). (B) Centrilobular necrosis.*[131]

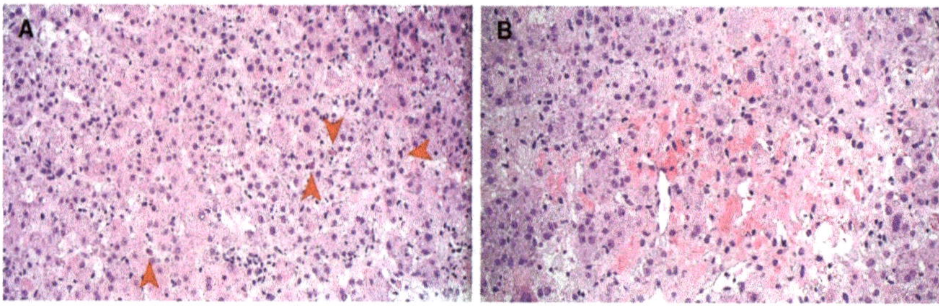

Can She Restart Nivolumab?

Yes, but very cautiously. You need to ensure she is still asymptomatic and responded to steroids or improved spontaneously—and only when her liver tests reduce to about 2-3x ULN (downgraded into the grade 1 territory). Typically, the clinical need for ICI is very compelling (e.g., active malignancy with limited treatment alternatives) to consider resumption in those with grade 3 or even grade 4 hepatotoxicity. But you may also want to consider switching ICI class if possible and the decision should always be made in collaboration with oncology. You just have to tread lightly with your eyes wide open.

Bringing It Together

This is a typical case of ICI-related hepatocellular injury—a dramatic ALT elevation with a calm clinical picture. If the patient is stable and the bilirubin is low, watchful monitoring is safe and often effective. Steroids are reserved for rising enzymes or worsening clinical status. And perhaps most importantly, this isn't a one-way street: with careful recovery and collaboration, restarting immunotherapy is often possible, preserving cancer control without sacrificing the liver.

So, the next time you see an ALT of 400 in a patient taking an ICI, pause before reaching for prednisone. The liver may just be asking for a break, not a full-blown immune reset.

Case 3.15: The Infection That Tips the Balance

A 58-year-old man with a history of alcohol-related cirrhosis (MELD 17) presents to the ED with confusion, fever, and mild abdominal pain. He has had multiple prior admissions for hepatic encephalopathy and increased ascites but was doing reasonably well at home. He stopped drinking 6 months ago and had recently started lactulose again for mild confusion.

On arrival, he is febrile to 102°F, blood pressure is 96/58 mmHg, heart rate is 112, and oxygen saturation is 95% on room air. He appears somnolent but arousable. His abdomen is distended with shifting dullness but no rebound or guarding.

Labs show: WBC 13.4 × 10^9/L; Creatinine 2.1 mg/dL (baseline 1.0); Total bilirubin 6.8 mg/dL; INR 1.9; ALT 56 IU/L; AST 88 IU/L; Sodium 131 mmol/L; Lactate 4.2 mmol/L. A diagnostic paracentesis reveals 580 neutrophils/mm^3 in ascitic fluid. Blood cultures and urine cultures are sent, and antibiotics are started.

Over the next 12 hours, he requires escalating vasopressor support and is transferred to the ICU. The admitting team notes that he is likely developing acute-on-chronic liver failure.

Know your guidelines!

1. What is the definition of acute-on-chronic liver failure (ACLF), and how does it differ from simple decompensated cirrhosis?
2. What are the most common triggers of ACLF?
3. How should this patient be managed acutely?
4. When is liver transplant indicated in this setting?

Case 3.15: What do the guidelines say?

Source: ACG 2022 Acute-on-Chronic Liver Failure Clinical Guidelines [132]

This is a classic presentation of ACLF—a patient with pre-existing cirrhosis or chronic liver disease, who suffers an acute insult, in this case a serious infection, and rapidly spirals into multi-organ dysfunction. The distinction between a routine hepatic decompensation and ACLF isn't just semantic—it's prognostic and often lifesaving. ACLF is potentially reversible but carries a much higher short-term mortality, requires intensive support, need for liver transplant and palliative care consultation for those not responding to therapy.[133]

Infection is the most common trigger for ACLF. Think about SBP or common sources like UTI or pneumonia

The ACG guideline frames ACLF as a distinct clinical syndrome marked by systemic inflammation, acute organ failures, and often poor outcomes. The most common trigger for this unfortunate cascade is infection, especially spontaneous bacterial peritonitis (SBP) or sepsis from common sources like urinary tract infections or pneumonia.

As an aside, we want to send a special shout-out to Dr. Jasmohan Bajaj, first author of the ACG ACLF guideline, for his tremendous work over the years advancing the science of clinical hepatology care. It's hard to imagine anyone, anywhere, who is more knowledgeable and passionate about cirrhosis and its complications than Dr. Bajaj. Kudos to you, sir!

From Decompensation to ACLF: What Changes the Game?

This patient is febrile and hypotensive, with altered mental status, an elevated creatinine, and evidence of SBP. He has known cirrhosis but now presents with new and escalating organ failures: encephalopathy, renal dysfunction, and early circulatory collapse.

His labs show creatinine 2.1 mg/dL (baseline 1.0); INR 1.9; total bilirubin 6.8 mg/dL; WBC 13.4×10^9/L; and lactate 4.2 mmol/L.

His ascitic fluid has 580 PMNs/mm^3—consistent with SBP. According to standard diagnostic criteria, SBP is diagnosed (after secondary bacterial peritonitis has been ruled out) when the absolute neutrophil count in ascitic fluid is ≥250 cells/mm^3, regardless of culture results. A positive culture confirms the diagnosis, but is not required to start treatment. In this case, a PMN count of 580 is well above that threshold and mandates immediate empiric antibiotic therapy and intravenous albumin, as per guideline recommendations.

When ascitic fluid PMN count exceeds 250, you've pretty much got SBP. Start treatment even if culture is negative

This is not a "garden-variety" hepatic decompensation. It is ACLF, and the key is recognizing it early—because timing matters for both intensive care triage and potential transplant referral.

How ACLF Is Defined

There are 3 major ways to define and grade ACLF, depending upon where you practice on a global level, that are discussed in the ACG guidelines, as follows:

- NACSELD (North American Consortium for the Study on End-Stage Liver Disease), which is used in North America and endorsed in the ACG guidelines, defines ACLF as 2 or more extrahepatic organ failures in a patient with cirrhosis hospitalized for an acute decompensation. It considers shock, respiratory failure, renal failure (creatinine ≥2 mg/dL or need for dialysis), and grade 3-4 hepatic encephalopathy as the critical components.[134] ACLF is staged from NACSELD-ACLF 1 to 4, depending on the number of organ failures.
- EASL-CLIF-C (European Association for the Study of the Liver-Chronic Liver Failure-Consortium), which is more commonly used in Europe includes liver-specific markers (bilirubin, INR) and uses a broader organ failure model based on the CLIF-C OF score.[135] While useful, it is more complex and less commonly used in U.S. practice.
- APASL (Asian Pacific Association for the Study of the Liver (APASL) defines ACLF in terms of level of acute hepatic decompensation in a patient with chronic liver disease without

requirement of extrahepatic organ failure (e.g. acute exacerbation of chronic hepatitis B).[136] This definition is not as commonly used in the Western Hemisphere.

Our patient, by NACSELD, likely meets criteria for at least ACLF-2: renal failure (Cr 2.1 mg/dL) and grade 3 HE (somnolence but arousable). He's also trending toward circulatory failure and getting close to ACLF-3. See **Table 3.9** for details comparing NACSELD to EASL-CLIF-C definitions

The key message: ACLF, according to NASCSELD, is not absolutely defined by the severity of liver disease per se, but by the number and type of organ failures that develop in the context of chronic liver disease.

Management: Time, Antibiotics, and Albumin

Start antibiotics as soon as possible for sepsis in ACLF since every hour matters and don't forget albumin for SBP

The cornerstone of management is rapid, broad-spectrum antibiotic coverage for suspected SBP and sepsis—ideally started immediately within recognition, since each hour delay in providing antibiotics in infected patients increases mortality, just as in other sepsis protocols.[137] To decrease mortality, this patient also requires albumin (1.5 g/kg on day 1, 1 g/kg on day 3) for SBP.[138]

Volume resuscitation should be judicious: enough to support perfusion, but not enough to provoke pulmonary edema or worsen ascites. Vasopressors may be needed early. Avoid nephrotoxins, hold diuretics, and monitor renal function closely. If shock or renal failure deepens despite these efforts, then early renal replacement therapy should be considered—especially if the patient is a transplant candidate.

Encephalopathy should be managed with lactulose and/or rifaximin; airway protection is considered if the patient becomes somnolent or progresses to grade 4 encephalopathy.

Organ support, not liver-specific treatment, is the mainstay—because the liver alone is often not the problem in ACLF. It's the systemic inflammatory response and the domino effect of organ failures that drive mortality.

What's the Prognosis—and Is Transplant on the Table?

ACLF is sobering: ACLF-2 carries a 41% 30-day mortality rate and it gets drastically worse as the number of organ failures increase.[139] But liver transplant may still remain a viable option, even in ACLF-3, if there is a chance of reversibility and no obvious contraindications.

The ACG guideline stresses early transplant center communication—not because every patient will be a candidate, but because late referral removes that option entirely. Frailty, active infection, poor functional status, and uncontrolled extrahepatic disease may all weigh against listing, but none should be assumed without discussion. If patients are not transplant candidates and not improving, then palliative care consultation should be undertaken for end-of-life care discussions with the family due to futility. Unfortunately, it is common that the patient may not be able to participate in those discussions due to the severity of the acute illness (encephalopathy, respirator, etc.).

Bringing It Together

This patient with cirrhosis, sepsis, renal failure, and encephalopathy is not just another decompensator. He's got acute-on-chronic liver failure, a syndrome defined by rapid-onset multi-organ failure in chronic liver disease, most often triggered by infection. The ACG guidelines ask us to recognize this early, treat it aggressively, support failing organs—and think fast about prognosis and transplant candidacy. If things are looking futile, then it's important to discuss end-of-life palliative care with the family and the patient if possible.

The infection tipped the balance. Our job is to recognize the fall and intervene before the rest of the system collapses. ACLF isn't just about the liver anymore—it's about time, triage, and survival.

Table 3.9. *Comparing NACSELD vs. EASL-CLIF-C Definitions of ACLF.*

Feature	NACSELD (*North America*)	EASL-CLIF (*Europe*)
Primary use	Adopted by ACG; widely used in U.S. clinical practice	Used in Europe; based on CANONIC study
Population	Hospitalized patients with cirrhosis and acute decompensation	Hospitalized patients with cirrhosis and acute decompensation, but includes more granular scoring
Definition of ACLF	$\geq$2 extrahepatic organ failures	$\geq$1 organ failure based on CLIF-C OF score
Organ systems assessed	4 systems: 1. Brain (grade 3-4 HE) 2. Kidney (Cr $\geq$2 mg/dL or dialysis) 3. Respiratory (mechanical ventilation) 4. Circulatory (vasopressor use)	6 systems: 1. Liver (bilirubin) 2. Kidney 3. Brain (HE) 4. Coagulation (INR) 5. Circulation 6. Respiration
Scoring/staging	ACLF-1 to ACLF-4 based on number of extrahepatic organ failures	ACLF grade 0-3 based on number/severity of failures across 6 organs
Prognostic utility	Predicts 30-day mortality; supports ICU triage	More detailed prognosis; used in research and transplant evaluation
Transplant guidance	Not formally built in, but used to prompt early referral	CLIF-C ACLF score can inform transplant candidacy and futility

Case 3.16: Renal Rebellion

A 64-year-old woman with a history of MASH cirrhosis and prior variceal bleeding presents with progressive fatigue and reduced urine output. She has been taking furosemide and spironolactone for ascites and reports recent nausea and poor oral intake due to a bout of gastroenteritis. She reports no fever or abdominal pain.

On exam, she appears volume depleted, with dry mucous membranes and is initially noted to have orthostatic hypotension. She is alert and oriented, without asterixis. Her abdomen is minimally distended but non-tender. There is no pedal edema.

Labs on admission show: creatinine 1.6 mg/dL (baseline 0.8); BUN 35 mg/dL; sodium 128 mmol/L; potassium 4.8 mmol/L; total bilirubin 3.1 mg/dL; INR 1.6; ALT 45 IU/L; AST 62 IU/L. Urinalysis shows no protein, no blood, a few hyaline casts, and no pyuria.

She is admitted to the hospital and started on intravenous fluids. Her creatinine rises to 2.3 mg/dL over the next 24 hours with a urine output of 300 cc despite IV albumin resuscitation. She no longer has orthostasis and has no known cardiac disease, and there is no evidence of obstruction on renal ultrasound.

Know your guidelines!

1. How is acute kidney injury defined in patients with cirrhosis—and when does it qualify as ACLF?
2. What are the steps to work up and manage acute kidney injury (AKI) in cirrhosis, and how is hepatorenal syndrome (HRS) diagnosed?
3. What treatments are recommended?
4. When should renal replacement therapy be considered?
5. What is the prognosis of ACLF in this setting of AKI?

Case 3.16: What do the guidelines say?

Source: ACG 2022 Acute-on-Chronic Liver Failure Clinical Guidelines[132]

In ACLF, renal dysfunction is often the first sign that the patient is about to unravel. This case captures a pattern many clinicians know all too well: a patient with cirrhosis, some mild stressor—gastroenteritis, diuretics, poor intake—followed by a rapid decline in renal function out of proportion to the clinical picture. What starts as "prerenal azotemia" can escalate into hepatorenal syndrome (HRS) or be the first organ failure in full-blown ACLF. The ACG guidelines remind us that kidney failure is both a marker of mortality and a modifiable factor—if caught and treated early. Let's go over this step by step.

Step 1: Recognize AKI in Cirrhosis—It's Not Just the Creatinine

In patients with cirrhosis, AKI is defined by the International Club of Ascites* (ICA) criteria—not by absolute serum creatinine cutoffs alone.[140] According to the ACG-endorsed definition, AKI is present when there's an increase in serum creatinine ≥0.3 mg/dL within 48 hours, or ≥50% from baseline within 7 days. Our patient has gone from a baseline of 0.8 to 1.6 mg/dL on admission and now to 2.3 mg/dL— meeting AKI Stage 2 (2.0-3.0× baseline). No hematuria, proteinuria, or obstruction is found.

> AKI is present when there's an increase in Cr≥0.3 mg/dL within 48hrs, or ≥50% from baseline within 7d

Importantly, even a "normal" creatinine can be misleading in cirrhotics, especially in older women with low muscle mass. That's why trending delta creatinine is more reliable than the absolute value.

Step 2: Determine if This ACLF or Not

This patient has cirrhosis, AKI, and hyponatremia—but is

* The "International Club of Ascites" sounds less like a panel of liver experts and more like a secret society where entry requires successfully performing a blind paracentesis in a moving vehicle. Still, they set the rules—so we salute them.

alert, normothermic, and currently hemodynamically stable. By NACSELD criteria, she has 1 organ failure—renal—and does not yet meet the threshold for advanced ACLF. However, she is at high risk for progressing to stage 2 ACLF if another organ tips (e.g., HE, shock, respiratory failure). According to the guideline, renal failure is both a major trigger and a key prognostic marker—with mortality sharply increasing as renal dysfunction deepens or multiplies.

Step 3: HRS-AKI—A Diagnosis of Exclusion

The ACG guideline recommends following a stepwise diagnostic and treatment pathway for AKI in cirrhosis:

1. Stop diuretics and correct volume depletion—usually with IV albumin, 1 g/kg/day (max 100 g/day) for 1-2 days.
2. Rule out infection, nephrotoxins, and obstruction.
3. If creatinine continues to rise despite volume resuscitation, and no other cause is found, HRS-AKI (formerly termed HRS type 1) is diagnosed.

In this case, the patient's creatinine rose from 1.6 to 2.3 mg/dL after adequate intravenous fluids, and her urine sediment is pretty bland. No obstruction is seen. Assuming sepsis and other insults are excluded, this is likely HRS-AKI. The guideline clarifies that you don't need to wait for creatinine to hit 5 or 6— the horse has left the barn at that point. Early diagnosis and treatment of HRS improves outcomes.

Step 4: Treat Early, Treat Right—Albumin + Vasoconstrictor

For stage 2 and stage 3 HRS-AKI, treat with a vasoconstrictor in combination with albumin. Vasoconstrictors are not recommended for stage 1 AKI (way too early) or stage 4 AKI (way too late). The preferred vasoconstrictor is terlipressin. If terlipressin is unavailable, then norepinephrine, which typically requires ICU administration by continuous infusion, would be recommended. Monitor for any ischemia-related events. Also, since these vasoconstrictors are given with IV albumin, you need to watch closely for hypoxia, pulmonary edema and volume overload.

The goal is not just to improve creatinine but to prevent progression to multi-organ failure. The response is assessed by improvement in creatinine after 3 days of therapy. If there is improvement, then continue for up to 14 days. Lack of improvement suggests either irreversible renal damage or underlying structural nephropathy and vasoconstrictor treatment should be stopped.

Step 5: What If Medical Therapy Fails? RRT and Transplant

If the patient is not a candidate for liver transplantation, then RRT may not be indicated

If renal function continues to decline, renal replacement therapy (RRT) may be required—but here's the critical point from the ACG guideline: RRT is not a bridge to nowhere. If the patient is not a candidate for liver transplantation, then initiating dialysis may prolong suffering without meaningful benefit.

For those who are transplant candidates, dialysis can stabilize the patient long enough to undergo liver transplant or simultaneous liver-kidney transplant (SLK) if renal failure is expected to be permanent. The guideline recommends considering SLK in patients with dialysis >6 weeks, CKD with GFR <30 mL/min, or kidney biopsy showing irreversible injury.

Bringing It Together

This case captures what the ACG guideline sees as the most common—and most modifiable—organ failure in ACLF: renal dysfunction. It starts subtly, often from dehydration, diuretics, or minor infections, but can rapidly progress to HRS-AKI, ACLF, and death. Early recognition, volume resuscitation, and vasoconstrictor therapy are critical. But so is stepping back to ask: Is this patient a transplant candidate? If the answer is yes, aggressive treatment and RRT may be lifesaving. If the answer is no, the focus may shift to palliation.

Case 3.17: The Incidentaloma

A 42-year-old woman is referred after undergoing a non-contrast abdominal CT for nephrolithiasis, which noted a 2.5 cm hypodense lesion in segment 8 of the liver. She has no history of liver disease, takes no medications, and has normal liver enzymes and synthetic function. She feels well and has no risk factors for hepatitis B or C, no alcohol use, and no family history of liver cancer.

The CT report describes a "low-attenuation lesion, non-specific in appearance." She is told she has a "liver mass," and understandably, she's worried.

Her primary care physician orders an AFP, which is normal, and refers her to GI for further evaluation.

Know your guidelines!

1. What is the initial approach to incidentally discovered liver lesions in asymptomatic, non-cirrhotic patients?
2. How does lesion size influence management decisions?
3. What imaging modality is best here?
4. When can you safely reassure and observe?
5. How should you counsel patients who are worried about "cancer" when most incidental liver lesions are benign?

Case 3.17: What do the guidelines say?

Source: ACG 2024 Focal Liver Lesions Guideline[141]

In the world of modern imaging, incidental liver lesions are everywhere. They show up uninvited on kidney stone scans, appendicitis work-ups, and trauma protocols. In a healthy, asymptomatic adult with no known liver disease, the overwhelming majority of these lesions are benign. Yet the language used to describe them—"liver mass," "indeterminate lesion," "hypodensity"—understandably provokes fear and anxiety in both the patient and the clinician. That apprehension often escalates into unnecessary referrals, repeated imaging, and, occasionally, a biopsy that never needed to happen. The ACG's guideline on focal liver lesions was written precisely to avoid that spiral—by helping us interpret incidental findings calmly, correctly, and with just enough precision to know when to step in and when to walk away. No doubt, these guidelines are key to know. It is important to know the basic gross anatomy of the liver segments shown below (**Figure 3.11**), since treatment can be impacted by the vascular supply.

Figure 3.11. *Segmental Anatomy of the Liver. Note that each liver segment receives inflow through branches of the portal vein (purple) and drains via branches of the hepatic vein (blue). The notable exception is segment 1, which drains directly into the inferior vena cava posteriorly.*[142]

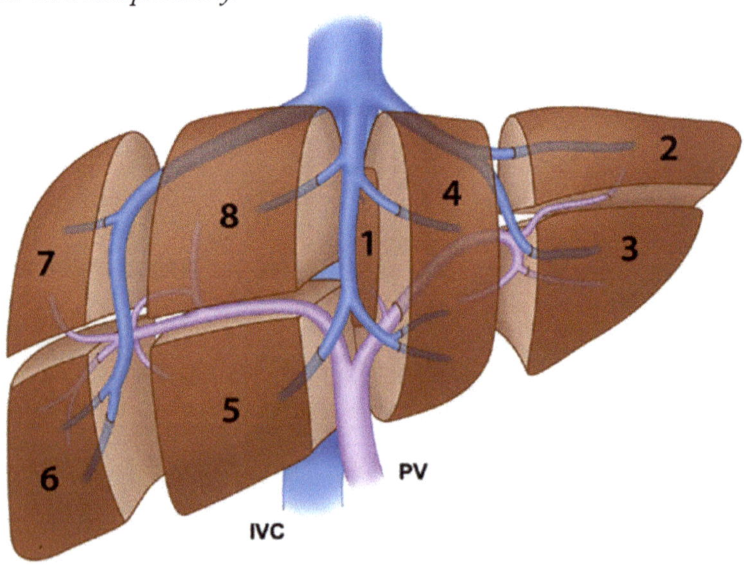

Understanding Risk Begins with the Host, Not the Lesion

The most important step in evaluating an incidental liver lesion is not to start with the imaging, but with the patient. Does this person have any underlying liver disease? Cirrhosis? Hepatitis B or C? Known cancer? In our vignette, the answer is no across the board. She has no viral risk factors, no alcohol use, no autoimmune or metabolic disease, no concerning medications, and a completely unremarkable liver panel. That alone moves her into a low-risk category, where the likelihood of hepatocellular carcinoma (HCC), cholangiocarcinoma, or metastasis is exceedingly small. This shift in perspective is vital: in a healthy, low-risk patient, an incidental lesion is far more likely to be a hemangioma, cyst, focal nodular hyperplasia (FNH; more on that later), or a small hepatic adenoma rather than something malignant.

> All things being equal, most incidentally found liver lesions are benign

The second question is size. This lesion is 2.5 cm, which places it in the "characterize once, don't panic" range. Lesions under 1 cm are often ignored entirely in low-risk patients. Lesions over 3 cm certainly deserve a closer look. But those in the 1-3 cm window, like this one, call for a single high-quality imaging study to define what we're looking at and decide whether it can be left alone or requires follow-up.

What Counts as a High-Quality Study?

The ACG guidelines emphasize that not all imaging is created equal. The CT that discovered this lesion was non-contrast, and while that's fine for finding kidney stones, it's essentially useless for fine liver characterization. What's needed is a multiphasic liver protocol study, ideally an MRI with contrast, including arterial, portal venous, and delayed phases. Hepatobiliary contrast agents like gadoxetate disodium can further refine the diagnosis, especially when distinguishing FNH from hepatic adenoma. A triple-phase CT is acceptable if MRI is unavailable or contraindicated, but the key is to specify the proper protocol—standard abdominal CT won't cut it. If radiology doesn't hear "liver lesion protocol," they won't run the

Figure 3.12. *A classic hepatic hemangioma with nodular discontinuous centripetal enhancement.*[144]

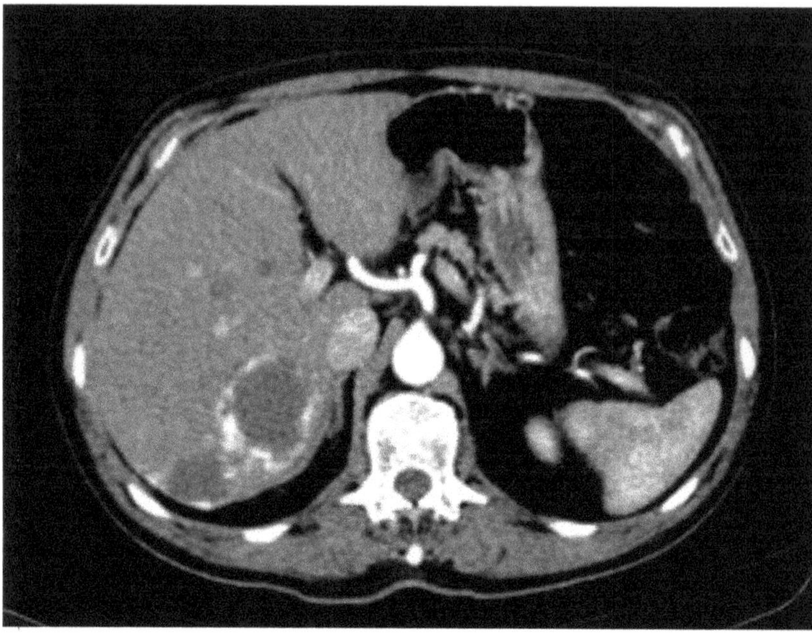

Figure 3.13. *Arterial-enhancing FNH with central scar, which is non-calcified. Note, if there were a calcified central scar, you should think about fibrolamellar hepatocellular cancer, not just benign FNH.*[145]

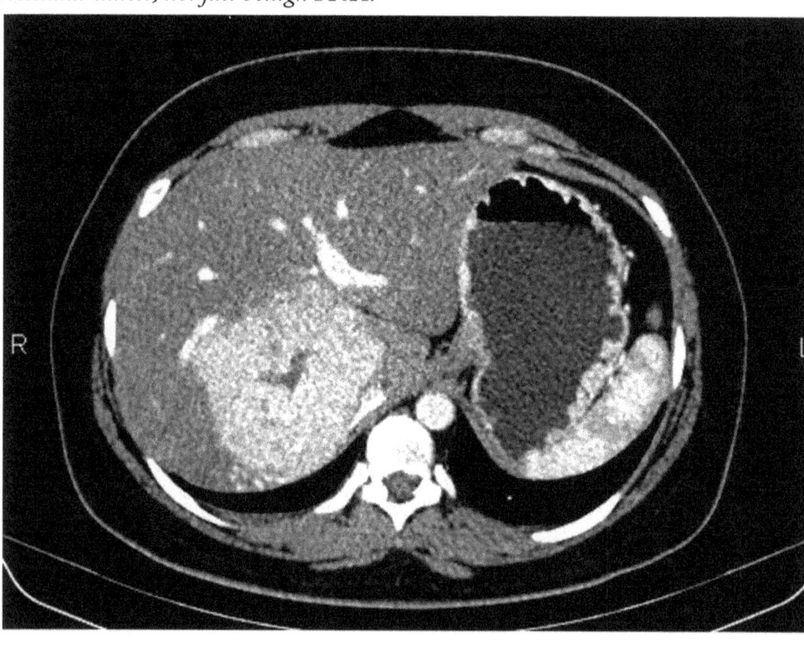

Figure 3.14. *MRI showing a 3 cm hepatic adenoma (arrows) in segment 5 which is hypointense on T1 pre-contrast with hyperenhancement on arterial phase (AP) and mild persistent enhancement on portal venous phase (PVP) of imaging. Biopsy in this case proved β-catenin hepatic adenoma. Thus, surgical resection was performed due to the propensity for transformation to HCC.*

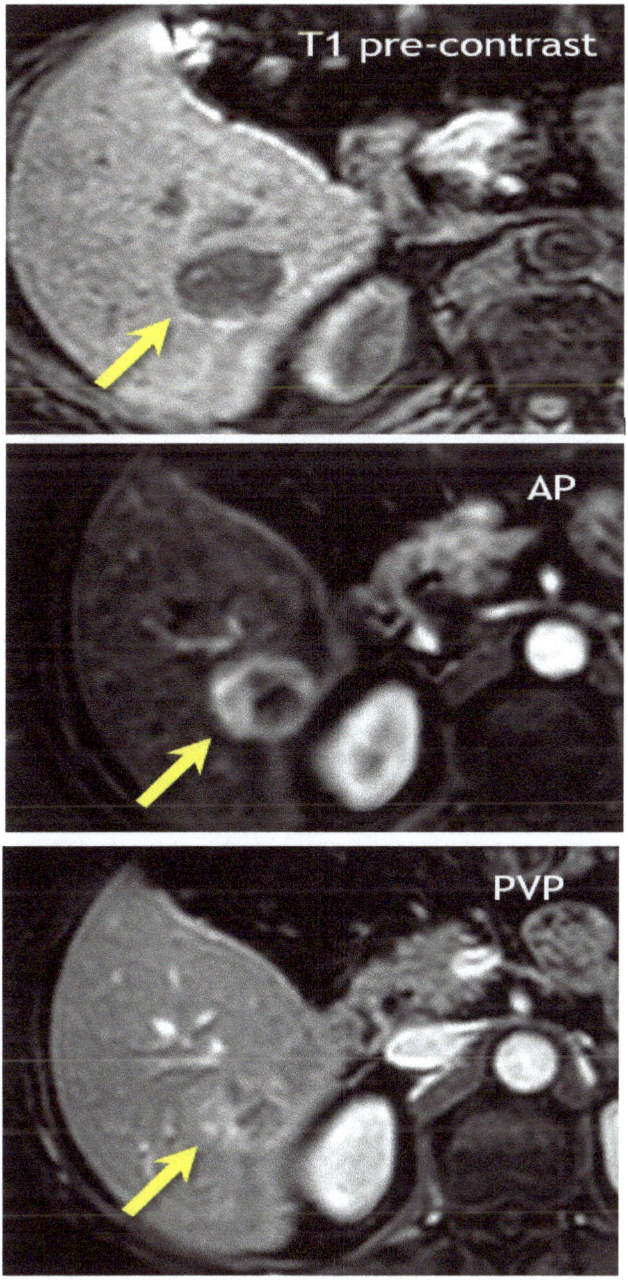

correct sequences. MRI has further advantages over CT by avoiding ionizing contrast and radiation. Nonetheless, whatever modality you choose, you should be aligned with local expertise to have the best quality interpretation since there hasn't been a statistically significant difference between MRI and CT in diagnosis of focal liver lesions.[143]

Get a multiphase MRI or triple-phase CT for incidental liver lesion >1cm found on non-contrast CT. MRI is typically preferred

Once this patient has a dedicated multiphasic MRI or CT, there's a good chance the lesion will declare itself. If it fills peripherally with progressive centripetal discontinuous nodular enhancement, it's a classic hemangioma (**Figure 3.12**). If it demonstrates homogeneous arterial enhancement with a non-calcified central scar and retains contrast on the hepatobiliary phase, it's almost certainly focal nodular hyperplasia (**Figure 3.13**). If it washes out, lacks a scar, or shows other atypical features, hepatic adenoma enters the picture (**Figure 3.14**), where a biopsy may be needed for clarification. But in the absence of risk factors and with a classic imaging pattern, a biopsy can be averted in the majority of cases like this one. For a refresher, check out the guideline, where you'll see an expansive set of algorithms which summarizes how to approach a focal lesion such as this.

There is no need for serial AFPs or long-term surveillance if the lesion remains stable for years. And critically, there is no need for biopsy unless the lesion grows, develops suspicious features, or the patient's risk profile changes.

By contrast, if the lesion grows, develops arterial enhancement with washout, or if the patient has new cancer elsewhere, the work-up shifts toward biopsy or multidisciplinary tumor board evaluation. But that's not the patient in this vignette.

The Art of Reassurance

For patients, the phrase "you have a liver lesion" is deeply unsettling. Many assume the worst, and Google or GPT is not their friend. This is where clear, confident communication is essential. It helps to say, "These are common and usually harmless. But based on your history and blood work, let's do one high-quality scan so we can tell more about what it is. In most people like you, it usually turns out to be something we can ignore." This reinforces the guideline's key point: not every lesion deserves a lifetime of follow-up.

Bringing It Together

This case captures one of the most common clinical scenarios in hepatology—and one of the most mismanaged. The ACG guidelines remind us to start with the patient's risk factors, not the radiology report. For lesions between 1-3 cm in low-risk patients, one good imaging study is usually enough to close the case. If it's a hemangioma or FNH, no follow-up is needed. And in almost all cases, biopsy is not the next step. The goal is to get the diagnosis right, not to chase every shadow in the liver with a needle.

In short: One scan, well chosen, can save a patient from months of worry—and save a clinician from a long string of unnecessary work-ups. That's what guidelines are for.

Case 3.18: The Cirrhotic Liver Nodule

A 58-year-old man with a history of hepatitis C-related cirrhosis is undergoing routine HCC surveillance. He was treated with direct-acting antivirals 2 years ago and achieved a sustained virologic response. His liver disease remains compensated (Child-Pugh A), and he has no history of variceal bleeding, encephalopathy, or ascites.

His most recent surveillance ultrasound shows a 2.4 cm hypoechoic lesion on ultrasonography (**Figure 3.15**). He is asymptomatic and his liver panel is stable. AFP is 9 ng/mL. His primary care provider refers him for further evaluation.

Figure 3.15. *Hepatic ultrasound shows 2.4 cm hypoechoic lesion (arrow).*[146]

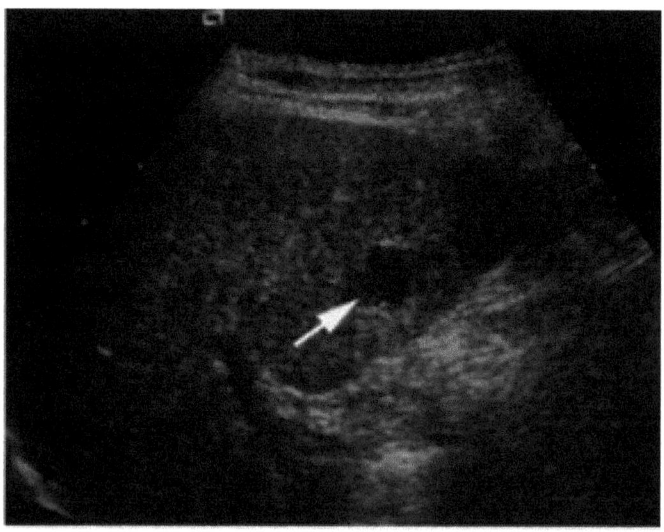

Know your guidelines!

1. How should a new lesion in a cirrhotic liver be approached?
2. What role does LI-RADS play here?
3. When can HCC be diagnosed noninvasively?
4. How does lesion size and imaging guide management?

Case 3.18: What do the guidelines say?

Source: ACG 2024 Focal Liver Lesions Guideline[141]

In a patient with cirrhosis, a new focal liver lesion should always be treated with a presumption of malignancy—until imaging proves otherwise. This is a completely different calculus from the healthy liver "incidentaloma" discussed earlier, where we start with the assumption the lesion is benign. Cirrhosis transforms the diagnostic landscape: nodules in this setting are common, but so is HCC, and delays in diagnosis can mean the difference between curative therapy and palliative care. The ACG Focal Liver Lesions Guideline doesn't get into HCC and instead refers readers to the AASLD practice guidance on HCC.[147] But since you are bound to run into a case like this, we thought we would hit you up with some bonus coverage including tips from the European Association for the Study of the Liver.[148] Our 58-year-old patient, with a compensated cirrhotic liver and a new 2.4 cm lesion, lands squarely in the zone where early detection matters most. Here we will simplify some key points from those liver society guidelines.

Focal liver lesion in cirrhosis = Start with assumption this might be cancer

First Steps: Confirm It's a Lesion, Then Characterize It Properly

Ultrasound is an excellent screening tool, but it is not a diagnostic one. When a nodule is seen on surveillance ultrasound in a cirrhotic liver, the next step is not biopsy or AFP—it's dedicated, multiphasic, contrast-enhanced imaging with either MRI or CT. But MRI is usually preferred for its higher sensitivity, especially for smaller lesions like this 2.4 cm nodule.

The key is to request a liver-specific multiphasic study, including arterial, portal venous, and delayed phases. Imaging must be protocol-driven, with sequences optimized for the liver—not just a generic abdominal scan. This is essential, because the diagnosis of HCC in cirrhotics is now made radiographically, based on hallmark vascular behavior.

Once the multiphasic MRI or CT is done, it should be interpreted using the LI-RADS (Liver Imaging Reporting and Data System) classification, which standardizes how liver lesions in at-risk patients are assessed and reported. LI-RADS categories range from LR-1 (definitely benign) to LR-5 (definitely HCC). An indeterminate lesion (LR-3) may be monitored, while LR-4 (probably HCC) may prompt closer imaging or even treatment in some centers. A lesion is labeled LR-5—definite HCC—if it shows arterial phase hyperenhancement with washout in the portal venous or delayed phase and is ≥1 cm (See **Figure 3.16**).

> Use LI-RADS to classify liver nodules in cirrhosis, as follows:
> LR-1 = Definitely benign
> LR-2 = Probably benign
> LR-3 = Unclear, monitor
> LR-4 = Probably HCC
> LR=5 = Definitely HCC

Figure 3.16. *LI-RADS Classification.100 LR-NC (non-categorizable), LR-1 (definitely benign), LR-2 (probably benign), LR-3 (intermediate probability of malignancy), LR-4 (probably HCC), LR-5 (definitely HCC), LR-M (probably or definitely malignant, not HCC specific), LR-TIV (tumor in vein).*[149]

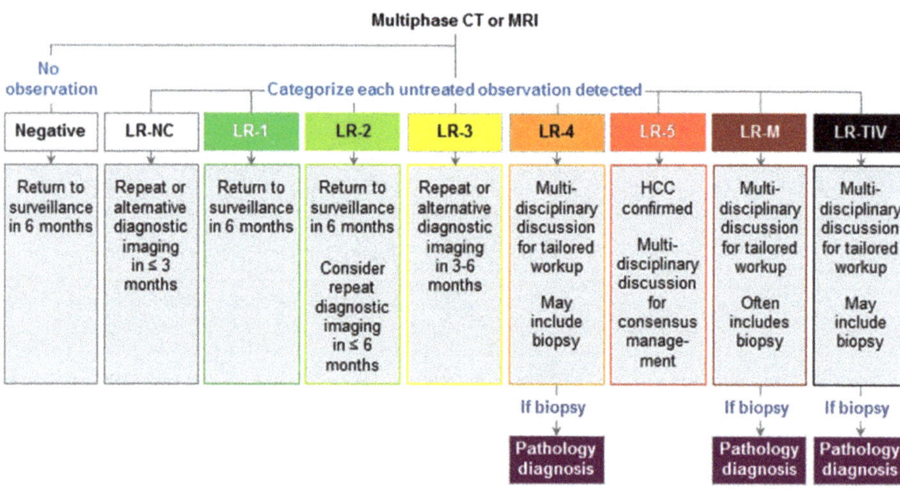

In our case, if the 2.4 cm lesion shows classic enhancement behavior—bright in the arterial phase, darker (washout) in the portal venous phase, with or without a pseudocapsule—then it qualifies as HCC by imaging alone. No biopsy is required. That diagnosis can be used to trigger liver transplant listing, surgical resection, or local ablative therapy depending on the patient's liver function and tumor burden.

The Role (and Risk) of Biopsy

The guideline is clear: biopsy is not the preferred first step in a cirrhotic patient with a new lesion. If the lesion is < 1 cm, you monitor it with repeat imaging every 3-6 months. If it's ≥1 cm, then management depends on the LI-RADS category Indeterminate lesions (LR-3 or LR-M) may warrant short-interval follow-up or biopsy, but even then, the decision still needs to go through a multidisciplinary tumor board discussion. Why so much caution around biopsy? Because the risk of tumor seeding along the needle tract—though small—is not zero. In fact, tumor seeding makes this stage 2 curable HCC into a stage 4 metastatic tumor. Also importantly, you don't need pathology to treat when the imaging tells the story. In experienced hands, imaging has a specificity >95% for HCC when classic criteria are met.[150]

> If 1 cm or greater lesion then manage according to LI-RADS classification

> Don't biopsy a LR-5 lesion since it is definite HCC and liver biopsy has risk of complications including tumor seeding

AFP and Other Biomarkers: Supplemental, Not Definitive

AFP can be helpful in some contexts, but in isolation it's only 49% sensitive with a specificity of 88% for HCC.[151] Thus, in this case, an AFP of 9 ng/mL doesn't move the needle in either direction. However, if the AFP was > 1,000 ng/mL after treatment, then that is an absolute contraindication to transplantation. Such a high AFP means that there's already vascular invasion and pretty much certain to have subsequent post-transplant HCC recurrence. In fact, the AFP needs to get below 500 ng/mL after treatment, to even be eligible for a liver transplant in the United States.[146] Moreover, in this context, the European guidelines consider AFP > 400 ng/mL a strong relative contraindication to transplant listing.[147]

Management Depends on Stage, Not Just Diagnosis

Once a lesion is classified as LR-5 HCC, the next step is staging. Patients with single tumors ≤5 cm or up to 3 tumors ≤3 cm without vascular invasion or metastasis meet the Milan criteria for liver transplantation. Others may be candidates for

Milan criteria for liver transplant eligibility:

* Single tumor <5 cm
* Up to 3 tumors, each ≤3 cm
* No vascular invasion
* No mets

resection, radiofrequency ablation, transarterial radioembolization (TARE) or transarterial chemoembolization (TACE). The choice depends on liver function, portal hypertension, performance status, and local expertise—but it all starts with getting the imaging right. Ultimately, management decisions are best determined at multidisciplinary liver tumor meetings.

Bringing It Together

This is one of the most consequential vignettes in this entire chapter. In a cirrhotic liver, a nodule is cancer until proven otherwise—but thankfully, we now have the tools to prove it without a needle. There's a central role of high-quality, multiphasic imaging, interpreted through LI-RADS, in diagnosing HCC noninvasively. Deciding upon the optimal course of therapy for any significant lesion is best determined after discussion with a multidisciplinary team. If a lesion shows the classic vascular pattern, you don't biopsy it, you treat it. If it doesn't, you watch it—or, if it's worrisome or ambiguous, might even biopsy it. But only after you discuss it with a multidisciplinary team.

In the right patient, at the right time, with the right imaging, a 2.4 cm nodule isn't just a finding—it's a curable cancer. That's why this pathway matters.

Case 3.19: Solid and Vascular

A 35-year-old woman undergoes an MRI for vague upper abdominal discomfort. She has no history of liver disease, does not drink alcohol, and takes oral contraceptives. Her liver enzymes are normal, and she feels generally well.

The MRI reveals a 3.5 cm hypervascular lesion in segment 3 of the liver. It enhances briskly in the arterial phase and shows a central scar. There is no evidence of washout or capsule, and the lesion retains contrast on the hepatobiliary phase using gadoxetic acid.

The radiologist suggests this may represent FNH, but hepatic adenoma cannot be ruled out.

Know your guidelines!

1. What imaging features help distinguish FNH from hepatic adenoma?
2. When is biopsy indicated here?
3. How does lesion size and subtype affect management?
4. What lifestyle modifications are recommended?
5. When is resection appropriate?

Case 3.19: What do the guidelines say?

Source: ACG 2024 Focal Liver Lesions Guideline[141]

The liver loves to surprise us with vascular nodules—often in young women who are otherwise healthy, asymptomatic, and found while imaging something else entirely. When a hypervascular lesion shows up on MRI, the differential diagnosis narrows quickly, but not completely. The primary contenders are FNH and hepatic adenoma—2 lesions that share certain demographic and imaging features, but diverge sharply in terms of management. This vignette sits at the heart of the ACG guideline's section on solid, non-malignant lesions in the non-cirrhotic liver, and offers a clear opportunity to work through the decision-making process the right way—imaging-first, biopsy-last.

Hypervascular liver lesion on MRI in a young woman on OCP? Think FNH vs hepatic adenoma

FNH and Hepatic Adenoma: The Right Lesions, the Right Context

FNH and hepatic adenoma are the 2 most common solid hepatic lesions in women of reproductive age without underlying liver disease.

FNH is considered a benign hyperplastic response to a congenital arterial malformation. It's not a neoplasm, doesn't bleed, doesn't become malignant, and almost never needs intervention. Hepatic adenomas, by contrast, are true neoplasms, derived from hepatocytes, with the potential for hemorrhage and malignant transformation, particularly in larger or certain molecular subtypes. Distinguishing between the two is essential, and the ACG guidelines underscore the primacy of imaging in doing so.

FNH is benign. Hepatic adenoma has potential for malignant transformation. Big difference!

Imaging Features: The Central Role of Contrast Behavior

This patient's lesion is 3.5 cm, shows arterial phase hyperenhancement, has a central scar, and—critically—retains contrast on the hepatobiliary phase after gadoxetate disodium administration.

These findings are essentially diagnostic of FNH. The central scar, a hallmark of FNH, may not always be visible on ultrasound or CT but is typically seen on MRI. Most importantly, FNH expresses organic anion-transporting polypeptides (OATPs) and therefore takes up and retains hepatobiliary contrast, remaining isointense or hyperintense on the delayed hepatobiliary phase.

FNH classically retains hepatobiliary contrast after gadoxetate-enhanced MRI. Hepatic adenomas do not

By contrast, hepatic adenomas lack bile ducts and do not retain hepatobiliary contrast—they appear hypointense on the delayed phase. Adenomas may show arterial enhancement as well, but they often wash out or demonstrate more heterogeneous enhancement, particularly in inflammatory or β-cateninmutated subtypes. Some may have internal fat or hemorrhage, which can further help distinguish them.

Thus, this patient's lesion meets classic imaging criteria for FNH, and no biopsy is needed. The ACG guidelines are clear: when imaging features are diagnostic, particularly when using hepatobiliary contrast, observation is not needed either.

When to Biopsy? Only When Imaging Fails You

Biopsy should not be the first reflex when a liver lesion is discovered. The ACG guidelines reserve biopsy for cases where imaging is inconclusive, or where features are atypical for both FNH and adenoma. If the lesion does not show typical behavior, or if it fails to enhance normally, or if hepatobiliary phase imaging is indeterminate, then biopsy may be appropriate—ideally after discussion in a multidisciplinary setting.

Importantly, if the diagnosis is hepatic adenoma with an uncharacteristic appearance or there are imaging features that are concerning for malignant transformation, then a biopsy can help determine molecular subtype, which directly informs management. β-catenin-activated adenomas carry

If imaging suggests hepatic adenoma with uncharacteristic appearance or concern for malignant transformation, then biopsy can screen for beta-catenin-activated disease, which has highest risk the highest risk of malignant transformation and are generally resected regardless of size, while hepatocyte nuclear factor—1α-mutated and inflammatory subtypes may be observed if smaller and asymptomatic.[152]

Management of Hepatic Adenoma Depends on Size, Subtype, and Symptoms

Had this lesion been an adenoma, its 3.5 cm size would have placed it in the "gray zone." The ACG guideline recommends that adenomas <5 cm in size without high-risk features may be managed conservatively with lifestyle modification and monitoring. That is, discontinuation of oral contraceptives, weight loss in patients living with obesity to decrease potentially stimulating estrogen, and repeat imaging in 6-12 months to monitor for changes in size.

Hepatic adenoma >5cm, any lesion with beta-catenin mutation or any lesion in male patient should be resected

Adenomas ≥5 cm warrant greater caution. These are more likely to bleed, particularly during pregnancy, and may harbor malignant potential. Resection is generally advised for lesions >5 cm, lesions that grow despite hormonal withdrawal, any β-catenin–mutated adenoma or any male with an adenoma, regardless of size due to increased risk of malignant transformation.[153]

FNH: Benign and Boring (In a Good Way)

The beauty of FNH is that once you know it's FNH, you're done. No follow-up, no lifestyle restrictions, no risk of bleeding or cancer. The ACG guidelines do not recommend serial imaging, oral contraceptive cessation, or any form of intervention unless the lesion is symptomatic (which is rare). The only real risk is misdiagnosing an adenoma or HCC as FNH—another reason why proper, protocol-driven imaging is key.

Bringing It Together

This case is a perfect reminder that not all liver masses are worrisome. A 3.5 cm arterial-enhancing lesion with a central scar that retains hepatobiliary contrast is diagnostic for FNH, and requires no biopsy and no treatment. The ACG guidelines champion a confident, imaging-based approach to these cases, sparing patients unnecessary procedures and sparing clinicians from over-investigation.

The liver may be solid and vascular—but in this case, it's just doing something common, benign, and completely manageable. The trick is knowing when to walk away from the work-up—and when not to reach for the needle.

Case 3.20: Gestational anxiety

A 23-year-old woman, 31 weeks into her first pregnancy, is referred for evaluation of abnormal liver tests, mild nausea, and early satiety. She reports fatigue and some nonspecific skin changes but denies jaundice, pruritus, fever, or abdominal pain. She's still eating—just in smaller portions—and has gained 4 lbs over the past 2 weeks.
Her obstetrician is wondering if she needs to be admitted. The patient is anxious, too.

Vitals: Temp 98.8°F; BP 102/64 mmHg; HR 96 bpm.

Exam: Bilateral palmar erythema, a few spider angiomas, gravid abdomen with trace pitting edema. No hepatomegaly or abdominal tenderness.

Labs: ALT 20 IU/L, AST 19 IU/L, total bilirubin 1.0 mg/dL, ALP 228 IU/L, GGT 25 IU/L; albumin 3.4 g/dL; BUN 6 mg/dL; creatinine 0.4 mg/dL; glucose 92 mg/dL; WBC 4.5×10^9/L; hemoglobin 11.4 g/dL; platelets 204×10^9/L.
Serum bile acids: Normal
Autoantibodies: AMA and ANA negative
Ultrasound: Normal liver, gallbladder, and spleen

Know your guidelines!

1. Do these lab abnormalities represent a physiologic change in pregnancy or something pathologic?
2. Should this patient be admitted?
3. What conditions should be ruled out at this gestational stage?
4. How should she be monitored moving forward?

Case 3.20: What do the guidelines say?

Source: ACG Clinical Guideline: Liver Disease and Pregnancy[154]

When you're consulted on a pregnant patient, it's natural to feel a little on edge. You're thinking about the mother, the fetus, and—if we're being honest—yourself. But when you know what's normal, you can approach these cases with much more confidence. And in this case? This is a normal pregnancy. There's no need for hospital admission, and no further testing is required at this time. She should be followed expectantly by her obstetrician, and you can offer some much-needed reassurance.

This vignette illustrates many of the physiologic and lab changes that are normally expected in pregnancy.

Let's Break It Down

Her nausea and early satiety are most likely due to gastric compression from the growing uterus. She's adapted by eating smaller meals—and she's still gaining weight, which is a good sign for maternal-fetal health. Polyuria (though not mentioned here) is also common from similar mechanical pressure on the bladder.

> Cardiac output increases 40%-45% mostly due to plasma volume expansion during a normal pregnancy

Fatigue is another nonspecific symptom, but in this context, it likely reflects the increased energy demands of pregnancy. Cardiac output increases by 40%-45%, largely due to expanded plasma volume, which also explains her slightly low albumin, hemoglobin, BUN, and creatinine.[154] Hemodilution is a normal physiologic shift. Her modestly low blood pressure? That's due to systemic vasodilation. Later in gestation, BP often trends upward again.

> Palmar erythema and spider angiomas are due to elevated estrogen levels during a normal pregnancy

Palmar erythema and spider angiomas? Blame it on estrogen. Elevated ALP? That's the placenta talking. GGT stays normal. Note that her bilirubin is normal, so there's nothing to do here. However, any abnormal bilirubin in pregnancy (besides known Gilbert's syndrome) merits further work-up. AFP? That rises, too—courtesy of the fetus. Take a look at **Table 3.10** for some of the physiologic lab findings that you would expect in a normal pregnancy.

Table 3.10 *Normal Physiologic Lab Findings During Pregnancy.*

Lab test	Change in pregnancy
AST	None
ALT	None
GGT	None
Total bilirubin	None
ALP	Increase
AFP	Increase
Albumin	Decrease
Hemoglobin	Decrease
INR	None

So, deep breath: this patient is doing just fine. You can advise continued routine obstetric care, with no additional hepatology work-up needed at this time.

Case 3.21: Pregnant with Jaundice

A 31-year-old woman at 28 weeks' gestation presents with jaundice and RUQ discomfort. She reports nausea, low-grade fever over the past few days, fatigue, and anorexia. She frequently eats out, but has no recent travel or known sick contacts. Her only medication is a prenatal vitamin. She denies any over-the-counter medications, including acetaminophen, and takes no herbal supplements.

Vitals: Temp 99.3°F; BP 108/66 mmHg; HR 85 bpm.

Exam: Well-appearing with mild icterus. Abdomen is gravid but nontender, with no guarding or hepatomegaly.

Labs: ALT 742 IU/L; AST 620 IU/L; total bilirubin 2.7 mg/dL; ALP 231 IU/L, INR 1.0

Acetaminophen level: Undetectable

Ultrasound: Normal liver, bile ducts, gallbladder, spleen, and hepatic vasculature. Fetal gestation appears appropriate for age.

Know your guidelines!

1. What diagnoses should you be concerned about in a pregnant patient with jaundice and elevated transaminases?
2. Which key tests are needed to narrow the diagnosis?
3. How urgent is this situation, and does this patient need to be admitted?

Case 3.21: What do the guidelines say?

Source: ACG Clinical Guideline: Liver Disease and Pregnancy[154]

This is a "classic" case of viral hepatitis which shows a predominant hepatocellular pattern with elevated aminotransferases more so than a cholestatic pattern in comparison to the bilirubin and ALP (go back and review the work-up of abnormal liver tests for a refresher). Importantly, biliary obstruction has been ruled out—which is critical, given the increased risk of gallstones and related complications during pregnancy. When evaluating jaundice or abnormal liver tests in a pregnant patient, the first step is imaging, and ultrasound remains the preferred modality due to safety and reliability in this population.

Remember, viral hepatitis is the most common cause of jaundice in both pregnant and non-pregnant patients. Guidelines recommend a targeted viral hepatitis work-up, because several viruses pose unique risks during pregnancy—namely hepatitis A, B, E, and HSV.

Hepatitis A (HAV): Risky but Rarely Chronic

HAV can lead to gestational complications and preterm labor.[156] While it doesn't cause chronic disease, it has been linked to vertical transmission, including documented NICU outbreaks.[157] For neonates born to mothers diagnosed within 2 weeks of delivery, HAV immunoglobulin is advised to reduce transmission risk. Infection control matters here.

HAV immunoglobulin is given to the neonate if mother is diagnosed with HAV 2 weeks prior to delivery

Hepatitis B (HBV): Preventable Vertical Transmission

HBV is a key player in pregnancy. Without intervention, the vertical transmission risk can be as high as 90%, especially if the mother is HBeAg-positive and has a viral load >200,000 IU/mL. To reduce this risk, the most recent European clinical practice guidelines also recommend tenofovir as the antiviral drug of

HBV vertical transmission rate varies but can be as high as 90%

choice during pregnancy based upon safety and efficacy.[158] Moreover, tenofovir should ideally be started before the third trimester to prevent mother-to-child transmission and then continued long-term as needed, based upon the clinical scenario and patient choice.

Regardless of viral load, all infants born to HBV-positive mothers should receive active-passive immunoprophylaxis: HBV vaccine and HBV immunoglobulin within 12 hours of birth. This combination approach with antiviral therapy reduces the risk of transmission to 3%-8%.[159]

What About Hepatitis C (HCV)?

HCV has a vertical transmission risk of about 6%, which increases to ~11% if the mother is co-infected with HIV.[160] There's no role for C-section or avoidance of breastfeeding purely based on HCV status, unless there are open sores or cracked nipples.[161] While DAA therapy is highly effective, it's not yet approved during pregnancy, but treatment can be pursued in childhood if needed.

Overall vertical transmission of HCV is about 6%

Hepatitis E (HEV): Rare Here, But Don't Miss It

HEV has a fecal-oral route of transmission like HAV, but it's especially dangerous during pregnancy—particularly in South Asia, where symptomatic infection can rapidly progress to acute liver failure with high maternal and fetal mortality.[162] In the U.S., it's rare, but still worth considering. If suspected, check HEV IgM—early diagnosis is crucial if the clinical course worsens.

HEV hepatitis during pregnancy has worse outcomes for the mother and fetus

Herpes Simplex Virus (HSV): Low Bilirubin, High Stakes

HSV hepatitis is rare, but deadly if missed—with mortality approaching 75% if untreated.[163] It is easily misdiagnosed. In fact, most cases may be discovered at autopsy.[164] Clues include anicteric hepatitis with fever, respiratory symptoms, and classic mucocutaneous lesions, although these are not always present. HSV can progress rapidly to

HSV hepatitis can rapidly progress to anicteric acute liver failure. If suspected, then start empiric acyclovir immediately massive hepatic necrosis and ALF, even when bilirubin levels are only modestly elevated. So, if you even suspect HSV hepatitis, start empiric acyclovir immediately. Don't wait for HSV PCR or biopsy results to come back—because by then, it might be too late. Biopsy (see **Figure 3.18**) will typically show nonzonal severe hepatic necrosis, but treatment can't wait for that confirmation.

Figure 3.18. *HSV Hepatitis. Liver biopsy showing the characteristic diffuse nonzonal severe acute hepatic necrosis.*[165]

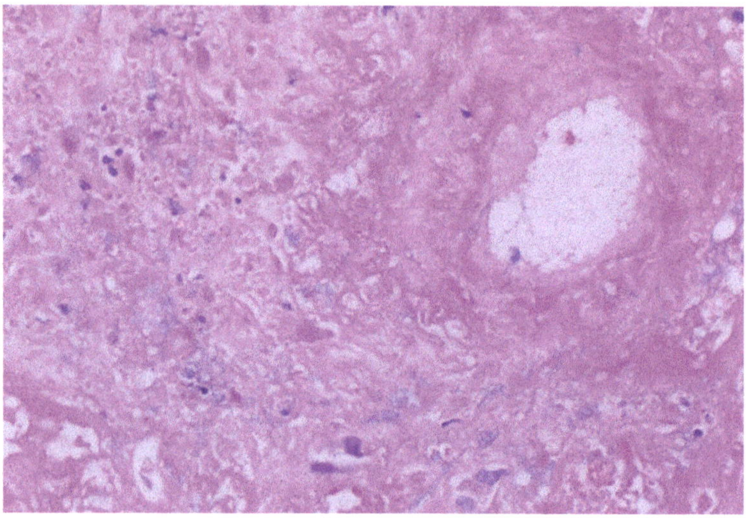

Bringing It Together

Pregnancy alters the physiology—but it doesn't exempt anyone from liver disease. In fact, some conditions (like HEV and HSV) are even more dangerous in this population. When facing elevated liver enzymes or jaundice in a pregnant patient, always start with an ultrasound, rule out biliary obstruction, and then think viral.

Run the right viral panel, keep your clinical suspicion sharp, and don't delay empiric treatment when warranted. And remember—in pregnancy, what looks mild can tip over fast. This is one of those moments when timing matters as much as diagnosis.

Case 3.22: The Pacer

A 22-year-old nulliparous woman with twin pregnancy presents to the ED with 6 days of severe nausea and vomiting at 8 weeks' gestation. She tried to pace herself and ate small portions at a time, but she has been unable to tolerate her food. She still then tried to pace herself and drink small portions of clear liquids but now she "can't keep anything down." There has been no hematemesis, abdominal pain, diarrhea or vaginal bleeding. She has also been unable to take her prenatal vitamins due to the persistent nausea and vomiting and notes that she has lost 9 lbs recently. She is worried about the remainder of her pregnancy as she wants to attend NBA basketball games since she is a season ticket holder. The ultrasound was normal and due to heightened patient concern and her wishes, a liver biopsy was performed (**Figure 3.19**) after shared decision-making.

Figure 3.19. *Liver Biopsy.*[166]

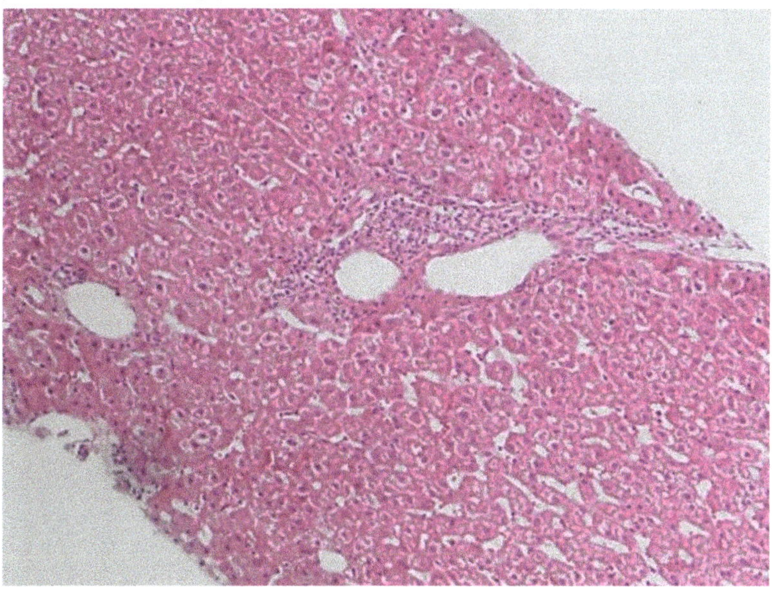

Labs: ALT 168, AST 124, TB 1.0, Potassium 3.4, Creatinine 1.2, Glucose 70, INR 1.0, WBC 7.9, Hemoglobin 14.9, Platelets 230. Urinalysis shows an increased specific gravity and is positive for ketones.

Know your guidelines!

1. What is the likely diagnosis in this patient with early pregnancy and severe nausea/vomiting?
2. How can liver enzymes be affected in this condition, and when should you be more concerned?
3. What risk factors increase the likelihood of this diagnosis?
4. What are the potential metabolic and nutritional complications of this condition?
5. When is hospital admission appropriate—and what treatments should be initiated?

Case 3.22: What do the guidelines say?

Source: ACG Clinical Guideline: Liver Disease and Pregnancy[154]

This is a classic case of hyperemesis gravidarum (HG). HG typically occurs in the first trimester and almost always resolves by 20 weeks' gestation. This patient's presentation is textbook—persistent nausea and vomiting, weight loss, and ketonuria with mild transaminase elevation. And yes, her twin pregnancy puts her at increased risk, as multiple gestations are a known risk factor.

Hyperemesis gravidarum occurs in first trimester and usually resolves by week 20 with supportive care

Liver enzyme abnormalities occur in more than half of patients with HG. Transaminases (ALT > AST) are usually elevated into the low hundreds, just like in this case. But unlike more ominous pregnancy-related liver diseases, liver injury is mild, and outcomes are typically excellent for both mother and fetus.[167] So, it's not surprising that her liver biopsy is normal (see **Figure 3.19**). Keep in mind that a liver biopsy is very rarely obtained and also should not be necessary in a suspected HG case.

Initial evaluation should focus on excluding other causes of nausea and liver enzyme elevation—particularly viral hepatitis, drug-induced liver injury, or other pregnancy-specific conditions. Once other causes are ruled out, treatment is supportive: intravenous fluids, antiemetics, electrolyte correction, and nutritional support if needed.[168] Patients like this one often require brief hospitalization, but they generally bounce back well with the right care. And yes—you can reassure her that she's still on track to make it to those Pacers games. Courtside dreams remain intact!

Shameless plug for the Indiana Pacers. After all, in 49 states it's just basketball. But in Indiana, basketball is a way of life!

Don't Confuse HG with ICP

One key pearl: don't confuse hyperemesis gravidarum with intrahepatic cholestasis of pregnancy (ICP)—the most common liver disease unique to pregnancy.

ICP usually presents in the second or third trimester with intense pruritus, often involving the palms and soles, before the onset of jaundice (which occurs in <25% of cases). There's typically no nausea or vomiting. The diagnostic test of choice is a serum bile acid level, with >10 μmol/L confirming the diagnosis. Levels >40 μmol/L are associated with increased risk of fetal distress, preterm labor, and even intrauterine demise, which is why close fetal monitoring and early delivery by 37 weeks is recommended.[169] The go-to treatment is ursodeoxycholic acid at 10-15 mg/kg of maternal weight. It lowers bile acids and improves outcomes.[170]

> Bile acid level > 40 μmol/L carries higher risk of fetal complications in ICP

Important to note—while maternal outcomes in ICP are excellent, fetal outcomes are the concern, and recurrence in future pregnancies is high. Patients should be counseled accordingly.

> UDCA decreases bile acid levels and improves fetal outcomes in ICP

Bringing It Together

This case highlights the importance of distinguishing what looks dramatic from what it actually is. While the labs may raise alarms, this is hyperemesis gravidarum—a benign, self-limited condition that can be managed supportively. In contrast, ICP carries significant fetal risk, and requires very different management.

When evaluating a pregnant patient with liver test abnormalities, timing matters. First trimester? Think HG. Second or third with itchy hands and feet? Think ICP. And don't forget to keep your viral and medication differentials in the mix.

With the right care, our patient will get back on her feet—and back to her courtside seats—in no time.

Case 3.23: Confused oil painter

A 31-year-old nulliparous oil painter at 37 weeks' gestation with twins presents with nausea, vomiting, epigastric pain, and jaundice for the past 2 days. She has no fever. Her husband adds that she has been acting confused and "not quite herself."

He became particularly concerned when he noticed her mixing oil paint colors directly on the canvas instead of on the palette—something she's never done before. Today, she's been lethargic and mostly sleeping, prompting him to bring her to the ED.

Labs: ALT 332 IU/L; total bilirubin 6.4 mg/dL; INR 2.1; creatinine 1.7 mg/dL; glucose 61 mg/dL; WBC 11.8 × 10^9/L; hemoglobin 12.1 g/dL; platelets 183 × 10^9/L.

Know your guidelines!

1. What diagnosis should be at the top of your differential in this late-pregnancy presentation with encephalopathy?
2. What features in this case are diagnostic clues?
3. What work-up should be initiated immediately?
4. What is the role of delivery in managing this condition?
5. What maternal and fetal risks should be anticipated?

Case 3.23: What do the guidelines say?

Source: ACG Clinical Guideline: Liver Disease and Pregnancy[154]

This is a classic case of acute fatty liver of pregnancy (AFLP)—a rare but life-threatening obstetric emergency. With an estimated incidence of about 5 per 100,000 pregnancies, AFLP is a condition you may not see often, but you definitely don't want to miss it when it shows up. It can rapidly lead to acute liver failure, renal dysfunction, coagulopathy, hypoglycemia, and in some cases, require urgent liver transplantation.[171,172]

AFLP is an obstetrical emergency as it can lead to acute liver failure and may require liver transplantation

This patient checks all the boxes: third trimester, twin gestation, nausea, vomiting, epigastric pain, jaundice, confusion, and laboratory signs of hepatic dysfunction (elevated transaminases, INR >2, bilirubin >5) along with hypoglycemia and renal impairment. The icing on the diagnostic cake? Her husband noticed she was "not quite herself"—a gentle way of noting early hepatic encephalopathy.

Pathophysiology: A Genetic Mismatch

AFLP is typically due to defects in intramitochondrial fatty acid oxidation, most notably involving long-chain 3-hydroxyacyl-CoA dehydrogenase (LCHAD). Many women with AFLP are heterozygous carriers of mutations affecting fatty acid metabolism, but the full clinical picture often unfolds when the fetus is homozygous for an LCHAD mutation.

In this setting, the fetus can't metabolize long-chain fatty acids, which build up and are shunted into the maternal circulation via the placenta. Mom's already reduced oxidative capacity gets overwhelmed, leading to microvesicular steatosis and liver failure.

About 20% of infants born to mothers with AFLP have homozygous LCHAD deficiency—so if you diagnose AFLP, genetic counseling and neonatal metabolic screening are part of the follow-up plan.

Diagnosis and Confirmation

The diagnosis is clinical and should be made promptly—don't wait for labs to worsen before acting. Fortunately, there have been clinical, laboratory, and imaging criteria, known as the Swansea criteria (**Table 3.11**), which may obviate the need for a liver biopsy.[173] If the diagnosis is still uncertain and time allows, a liver biopsy can show microvesicular steatosis on H & E stain (**Figure 3.20**); however oil droplets of microvescicular steatosis can be apparent with Oil Red O stain on a fresh specimen. In practice, however, biopsy is rarely necessary, as most cases are diagnosed based on history, labs, and clinical judgment. So, if the clinical picture is clear, treat first, confirm later.

Liver biopsy specimen in AFLP shows the characteristic microvesicular steatosis

Table 3.11. *Swamsea Criteria for Diagnosis of AFLP.*[172]

Six or more criteria required in the absence of another cause
Vomiting
Abdominal pain
Polydipsia/polyuria
Encephalopathy
Elevated bilirubin >14 µmol/l
Hypoglycemia <4 mmol/l
Elevated urea >340 µol/l
Leukocytosis >11x10^6/l
Ascites or bright liver on ultrasound scan
Elevated transaminases (AST or ALT) >42 IU/l
Elevated ammonia >47 µmol/l
Renal impairment; creatinine >150 µol/l
Coagulopathy; prothrombin time >14s or APPT >34s
Microvesicular steatosis on liver biopsy

Figure 3.20. *Microvesicular steatosis seen on H & E stain. Diffuse "foamy" hepatocytes with cytoplasmic microvesicular steatosis (arrows).*[174]

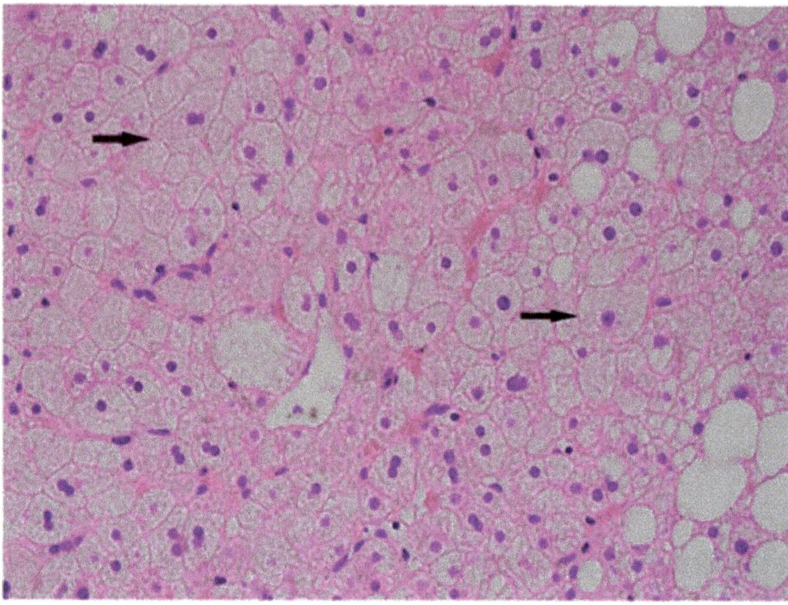

Act Fast—AFLP Can Spiral Quickly

> AFLP can have rapid deterioration. Prompt delivery is essential with ICU-level care. Urgent liver transplant evaluation could also be needed post-partum

Time matters in acute fatty liver of pregnancy (AFLP). This condition can deteriorate rapidly, and the risk to both mother and fetus is high. That's why prompt delivery is essential, along with ICU-level supportive care. But delivery doesn't guarantee recovery. The mother may still worsen post-partum, and if liver function doesn't improve quickly, she should be referred urgently for liver transplant evaluation.

And it doesn't end with mom. If the newborn has LCHAD deficiency, there's a real risk for life-threatening fasting-induced, nonketotic hypoglycemia in the first few months of life. So, the infant also needs metabolic screening and careful monitoring.

The risk of AFLP recurrence in future pregnancies is not well-defined, but appears to be low. That said, many women who survive a severe episode of AFLP are understandably hesitant to get pregnant again.

While We're Here: Preeclampsia, Eclampsia, and HELLP

Other liver-related pregnancy complications also deserve your attention—particularly preeclampsia, eclampsia, and HELLP.

- Preeclampsia is defined as SBP ≥ 140 or DBP ≥ 90 with proteinuria, typically after 20 weeks' gestation.
- Eclampsia is preeclampsia plus grand mal seizures.

These conditions can cause significant hepatic injury, often due to hepatic vasoconstriction, sinusoidal fibrin deposition, and even hepatic hematoma or rupture—which causes RUQ pain from Glisson's capsule stretch.[175] In these cases, the goal is to stabilize the mother and, if possible, get her to 34 weeks gestation for optimal fetal outcomes.[176] However, there is no benefit to continuing beyond 36 weeks, and delivery is recommended at that point regardless of maternal or fetal status.[177]

Delivery is recommended after 36 weeks with preeclampsia/eclampsia (if the patient is stable enough to wait until then)

Don't Miss HELLP Syndrome

HELLP—Hemolysis, Elevated Liver enzymes, Low Platelets—complicates up to 20% of preeclampsia/eclampsia cases. In addition to the expected AST/ALT elevation, you'll often see:

- Microangiopathic hemolytic anemia (↑ LDH, ↓ haptoglobin, ↑ indirect bilirubin)
- Thrombocytopenia

Histologically, HELLP is marked by periportal hemorrhage, sinusoidal fibrin deposition, and focal ischemic necrosis—a direct reflection of the underlying vascular injury (**Figure 3.21**).

HELLP has an increased risk with hepatic rupture, so delivery is recommended sooner than in preeclampsia. Don't wait until 36 weeks in HELLP and try to deliver as soon as 34 weeks

If you're dealing with sudden and severe abdominal pain and acutely worsening anemia, think hepatic infarction with rupture or subcapsular hematoma—a rare but devastating complication of HELLP. Unlike preeclampsia, where you might wait until 36 weeks, in these cases, deliver as soon as

Figure 3.21. *HELLP Syndrome Causing Hepatic Infarction. H & E stain showing massive hepatocellular necrosis and hemorrhage.*[178]

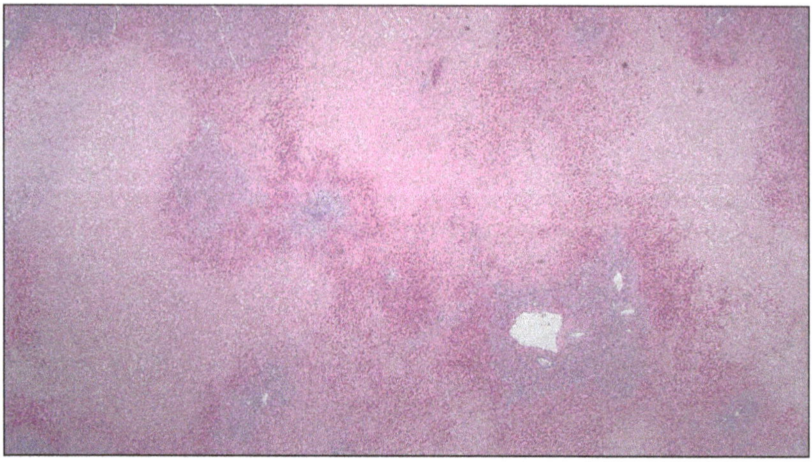

possible, optimally after 34 weeks. Treatment involves urgent delivery with angiographic embolization and/or surgery to control the bleeding. And because this can happen even after delivery, continued ICU-level monitoring is essential until the mother stabilizes. Urgent liver transplantation may be needed in severe cases (**Figure 3.22**).

Unfortunately, preeclampsia, eclampsia, and HELLP are not "one and done" diagnoses. Recurrence is common in future pregnancies, and patients should be counseled accordingly.

How can you tell the difference between AFLP vs HELLP?

It's often quite difficult to distinguish AFLP from HELLP, since there is a lot of overlap in laboratory tests and symptoms, such as nausea, vomiting and abdominal pain.[179] However, some clinical characteristics (as noted in the Swansea criteria in **Table 3.11**) can be quite telling of AFLP due to the ongoing liver dysfunction. Key features of AFLP include hypoglycemia, direct hyperbilirubinemia and confusion from encephalopathy. In contrast, HELLP is often characterized by more pronounced and progressive thrombocytopenia, indirect hyperbilirubinemia and increased lactase dehydrogenase from hemolysis, hypertension, proteinuria and a higher risk of disseminated intravascular coagulation. Since both conditions can wreak havoc with disastrous consequences for both the patient and fetus, you need to stay vigilant!

Figure 3.22. *HELLP Syndrome. Coronal CT scan showing marked peripheral hypoattenuation with central sparing consistent with massive hepatic infarction.*[178]

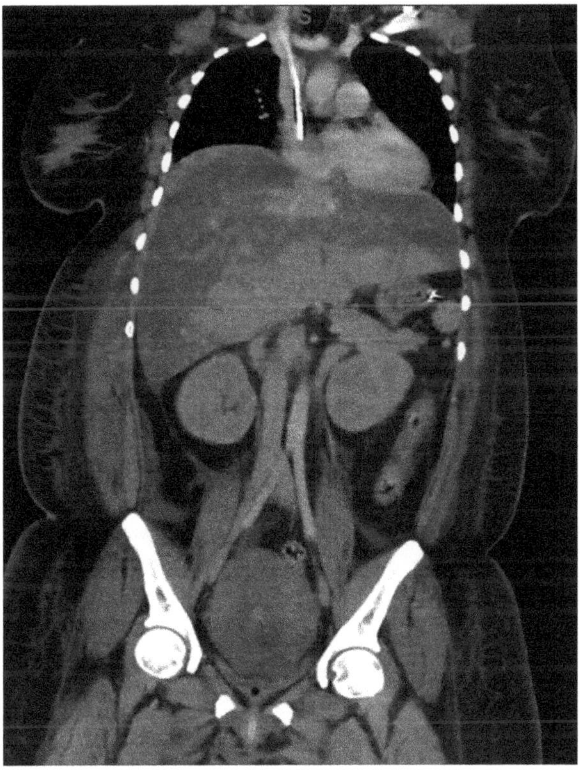

Bringing It Together

Pregnancy-specific liver diseases (**Table 3.12**) are rare—but when they happen, they demand fast thinking and decisive action. AFLP, HELLP, preeclampsia, and eclampsia can all present late in pregnancy with liver test abnormalities and overlapping symptoms. Your job is to recognize the pattern, anticipate the complications, and move quickly to protect both mother and baby.

AFLP is metabolic, HELLP is vascular, and preeclampsia/eclampsia are systemic—but they can all lead to acute liver injury, coagulopathy, and, in severe cases, multi-organ failure. The key takeaways?

- Don't wait on labs if the clinical picture is clear.
- Delivery saves lives, especially once you're past 34 weeks.
- And ICU care doesn't stop after the baby is born—not for these patients.

Table 3.12. *Liver Diseases Unique to Pregnancy.*[154]

Disorder	Trimester	Management
Hyperemesis gravidarum	First through 20 weeks	Supportive management
Intrahepatic cholestasis of pregnancy (IHCP)	Second/third	Ursodeoxycholic acid 10-15 mg/kg Early delivery at 37 weeks
Acute fatty liver disease of pregnancy (AFLP)	Third	Women with AFLP should be delivered promptly Infant should be monitored for manifestations of deficiency of long-chain 3-hydroxyacyl-coenzyme A dehydrogenase including hypoketotic hypoglycemia and fatty liver
Eclampsia, preeclampsia	After 20 weeks	After 36 weeks, women with severe preeclampsia should be delivered promptly
Hemolysis, elevated liver enzymes, low platelets (HELLP)	After 22 weeks	Delivery after 34 weeks Platelet transfusion to 40,000-50,000 cells/µl should be considered before delivery, especially if cesarean section is likely

Case 3.24: The Rusty Labs

A 52-year-old man presents to clinic for evaluation of fatigue and joint stiffness. He reports feeling "sluggish" for the past year, with low energy and intermittent dull pain in his hands and knees. He denies alcohol use and takes no medications aside from a daily multivitamin. He has no known liver disease and has never had abnormal labs in the past. His family history is notable for a brother with type 2 diabetes and a father who died of "liver problems," but no other known genetic conditions.

Routine labs reveal: ALT 48 IU/L; AST 42 IU/L; ALP 78 IU/L; total bilirubin 0.9 mg/dL. Ferritin is 684 ng/mL and transferrin saturation is 67%. His CBC, glucose, and creatinine are all within normal limits.

His primary care physician refers him to hepatology for possible iron overload.

Know your guidelines!

1. What are the first steps in evaluating elevated ferritin and transferrin saturation?
2. How do you distinguish hereditary hemochromatosis from other causes of iron overload?
3. What genetic testing should be ordered?
4. When is phlebotomy indicated?
5. What should patients be told about long-term management, prognosis, and family screening?

Case 3.24: What do the guidelines say?

Source: ACG 2019 Hereditary Hemochromatosis Guideline[180]

Here we have a middle-aged man with vague symptoms (fatigue, joint discomfort), slightly elevated liver enzymes, and unexpectedly high ferritin and transferrin saturation (TSAT). That lab combo—the high TSAT especially—is your first real clue that something's brewing in iron regulation. The ACG guidelines recommend a measured, stepwise approach to these cases, starting with repeat iron studies, followed by genetic testing when appropriate, and reserving imaging, biopsy, or therapy for those who truly meet diagnostic criteria for hereditary hemochromatosis (HH). Let's get into the details, step-by-step.

Step One: Repeat and Confirm

The first steps in evaluating elevated ferritin are to assess whether it's accompanied by elevated TSAT, and whether the findings persist. Ferritin is an acute-phase reactant—elevated in inflammation, infection, metabolic syndrome, alcohol use, and more—so a single high value can be misleading. But TSAT is more stable and more specific.[181] The ACG guideline uses a TSAT > 45% as the diagnostic trigger to investigate iron overload.

Remember that ferritin is an acute phase reactant, but TSAT is less susceptible to inflammation. If TSAT>45% and ferritin elevated look deeper and check genetics

In this patient, ferritin is 684 ng/mL and TSAT is 67%—both elevated. This is not diagnostic, but it's highly suggestive. The next step is not imaging or liver biopsy—it's HFE genetic testing, which should be ordered only after iron overload has been confirmed biochemically.

Step Two: HFE Genotyping—Who and What to Test

According to the ACG, those with TSAT >45% and elevated ferritin should undergo HFE gene testing. The test should look for the **C282Y** and **H63D** variants, which account for most genetically confirmed HH cases in people of Northern European descent.

If this patient is C282Y homozygous, the diagnosis of HFE-related hereditary hemochromatosis is confirmed. There is no need for liver biopsy at this stage if the ferritin is below 1,000 ng/mL, indicating very low risk for cirrhosis.[182] Also, the liver enzymes are only mildly elevated, and no other concerning features for advanced disease are present.

Step Three: Initiating Phlebotomy—When and How

The ACG recommends therapeutic phlebotomy for all patients with confirmed HH with iron overload (i.e., C282Y homozygosity or compound heterozygosity). The goals are to prevent organ damage—especially cirrhosis, diabetes, cardiomyopathy, and hypogonadism—and to relieve symptoms if present.

Induction phase phlebotomy is usually performed weekly or every other week until ferritin falls to 50-100 ng/mL. Each session typically removes 500 mL of blood, equivalent to ~250 mg of iron.

Once iron depletion is achieved, patients enter the maintenance phase, with phlebotomy every 3-4 months to keep ferritin between 50-100 ng/mL. Transferrin saturation is not used to guide therapy but is often tracked alongside the ferritin level.

Repeat phlebotomy q3-4 months and maintain ferritin 50-100. TSAT is not used to guide therapy

Step Four: Differentiating Primary HH from Secondary Iron Overload

The real-world challenge is that many patients—especially those with MASLD, excess alcohol use or chronic viral hepatitis—will have elevated ferritin but normal or mildly elevated TSAT. In these cases, iron overload is usually secondary, and HFE testing will be negative or non-diagnostic. Phlebotomy is not indicated for those patients unless iron overload is proven histologically or with imaging.

If ferritin elevated but not TSAT, consider:

* MASLD
* Alcohol
* Infection
* Inflammation

A helpful tip from the ACG guideline—isolated ferritin elevation without TSAT >45% almost never represents hereditary hemochromatosis, and these patients should not be reflexively tested or treated without further evidence.

Step Five: Counseling, Family Screening, and Prognosis

Once HH is diagnosed, the patient should be counseled that the condition is treatable, not curable, and that early intervention prevents complications. Phlebotomy is safe, inexpensive, and well tolerated in most patients, though mild anemia or symptomatic hypotension may occasionally occur.

HH is autosomal recessive. Be sure to screen 1st degree relatives appropriately

Because HH is autosomal recessive, first-degree relatives should be screened. For siblings of C282Y homozygotes, HFE testing is recommended, since they have a 25% chance of being homozygous themselves. For children, testing is usually deferred until adulthood unless clinical concern is present. Importantly, life expectancy is normal in patients treated before the development of cirrhosis or diabetes.[183] Some of the most commonly associated presenting symptoms—fatigue, cardiomyopathy, skin pigmentation, subtle transaminase elevations—often improve with therapy; however, diabetes, arthropathy, and hypogonadism tend to persist even after iron depletion.

Bringing It Together

This patient's presentation is a textbook example of how hereditary hemochromatosis often hides in plain sight—disguised as fatigue, joint pain, or "mildly abnormal labs." The guideline's algorithm is deliberate: confirm iron overload first (TSAT >45%, ferritin elevated), then proceed to HFE testing, and if C282Y homozygosity is found, begin phlebotomy without biopsy unless there are advanced findings.

Case 3.25: Ironclad Truths

A 61-year-old man with a history of cryptogenic cirrhosis is referred for evaluation of iron overload. He was diagnosed with cirrhosis 2 years ago based on imaging and transient elastography but has never undergone liver biopsy. He has no history of viral hepatitis, significant alcohol use, or metabolic syndrome.

Recent labs show: ferritin 1,512 ng/mL; TSAT 78%; ALT 52 IU/L; AST 67 IU/L; ALP 85 IU/L; INR 1.2. Platelet count is 118,000. HFE genetic testing reveals C282Y homozygosity.

He has no signs of decompensation and remains active, although he reports mild fatigue. An ultrasound performed 6 months ago showed a nodular liver and mild splenomegaly but no focal lesions and no ascites.

Know your guidelines!

1. How should C282Y homozygosity be interpreted here?
2. What is the role of liver biopsy in this setting?
3. When should HCC surveillance be initiated in HH?
4. Can iron depletion improve outcomes even after cirrhosis?
5. What's the long-term management plan?

Case 3.25: What do the guidelines say?

Source: ACG 2019 Hereditary Hemochromatosis Guideline[180]

In the real world, many patients with hereditary hemochromatosis don't come to attention during the early, asymptomatic phase. Instead, they show up already cirrhotic, often labeled as "cryptogenic" or misattributed to MASLD, with iron overload discovered only after a ferritin creeps above 1,000 ng/mL or an MRI flags hepatic siderosis. That's what makes this vignette so important: it illustrates the diagnostic and prognostic work-up of late-presenting HH, and how the management shifts once cirrhosis is established—even if iron is still accumulating.

This patient has C282Y homozygosity, a ferritin well over 1,000 ng/mL, TSAT of 78%, and a prior diagnosis of cirrhosis. While the genetics are ironclad, the presence of cirrhosis adds nuance to virtually every decision—from the role of biopsy to HCC surveillance and beyond.

C282Y Homozygosity + Cirrhosis = Probable HFE-Related HH

Remember that C282Y homozygosity is not, unto itself, diagnostic of HH. Also look for evidence of iron overload TSAT > 45% and elevated ferritin

C282Y homozygosity is the genetic signature of classical, autosomal recessive HFE hemochromatosis. On its own, it's not diagnostic—many homozygotes never develop clinically significant iron overload—but in the presence of elevated ferritin and TSAT >45%, and particularly in the absence of other clear causes of liver disease, the diagnosis of HH is confirmed. No further genetic testing is needed.

He's homozygous, he's iron-loaded, and he's cirrhotic. The big question now is—what next?

Liver biopsy is not required to diagnose HH if genetics and iron studies add up

Is a Liver Biopsy Still Needed? Sometimes—But Not Always

In most patients with confirmed HFE-HH and iron

overload, liver biopsy is no longer necessary. But the ACG guidelines carve out exceptions, particularly in patients with:

- Ferritin >1,000 ng/mL
- Concurrent risk factor for cirrhosis
- Clinical features of advanced fibrosis on physical exam, labs, or imaging

In this case, the patient is already diagnosed with cirrhosis, so biopsy won't change that. But if the prior diagnosis had been unclear on imaging without a stiffness measurement, a liver biopsy could still have value—either to confirm the stage or to detect overlapping etiologies (e.g., MASLD, alcohol, viral hepatitis, etc.). Importantly, biopsy can also quantify hepatic iron concentration, and when coupled with fibrosis staging, can help determine whether non-HFE forms of HH or iron-loading anemias should be considered (though rare in this setting). Newer MRI T2-weighted techniques have evolved and shown to be useful for estimating hepatic iron concentrations.[184]

Bottom line:
If cirrhosis is already established by imaging or elastography, and HFE-HH is confirmed genetically, biopsy is not required—but may be helpful if the picture is murky.

Ferritin >1,000 Increases the Risk of Harboring Cirrhosis

The risk of cirrhosis increases once ferritin >1,000

The ACG guideline highlights ferritin >1000 ng/mL as a key threshold: it's the level above which advanced hepatic fibrosis or cirrhosis is much more likely, even in patients with normal ALT and AST. Once cirrhosis is established—by biopsy, imaging, or noninvasive markers—the management shifts permanently, regardless of whether the patient undergoes phlebotomy. That means:

- Liver ultrasound with or without AFP every 6 months for HCC surveillance[148]
- EGD at diagnosis to screen for varices
- Lifestyle counseling to avoid alcohol, and to assess for other contributors to hepatic injury

- Remind the patient (as you initially told them at diagnosis) that they need to avoid vitamin C supplements (which can increase iron absorption) and avoid eating uncooked oysters (risk of *Vibrio* infection).

This surveillance does not stop once the iron is removed. The initial stage of disease at diagnosis should be used for HCC surveillance, even though phlebotomy can sometimes later reverse advanced bridging fibrosis or cirrhosis, as noted on subsequent assessments, such as elastography with normalization of ferritin and liver tests. This is a critical teaching point: phlebotomy improves outcomes, but it doesn't erase the HCC risk after the patient has initially reached cirrhosis.[185]

Phlebotomy does not eliminate the HCC risk after the patient has cirrhosis

Does Phlebotomy Still Help After Cirrhosis Has Set In? Yes, But...

Phlebotomy remains the cornerstone of treatment, even in patients with cirrhosis. The ACG guidelines recommend regular phlebotomy until ferritin falls to 50-100 ng/mL, unless anemia or clinical intolerance limits therapy. The benefits, even in late-stage HH, include:

Target ferritin of 50-100 with phlebotomy

- Stabilization or improvement of liver tests
- Potential reversal of early-stage fibrosis
- Prevention of further iron-mediated damage to heart, pancreas, joints, and pituitary

In some cases, particularly when anemia, CHF, or intolerance limits phlebotomy, iron chelation therapy (e.g., deferasirox) may be considered—but this is second-line, used only in those who can't be bled.

Bringing It Together

This patient's story happens more often than it should: the "cryptogenic" cirrhotic who was never fully worked up for iron overload. Now, with thrombocytopenia, a ferritin >1,500, and C282Y homozygosity, the diagnosis is no longer cryptic. It's hereditary hemochromatosis with cirrhosis, and that comes with a permanent commitment to HCC surveillance, regardless of how well he feels or how low his ferritin eventually goes.

Phlebotomy is still indicated in advanced bridging fibrosis or cirrhosis, and it still helps. The ship has sailed on preventing HCC, but it's not too late to steady the course, prevent further damage, and keep one eye firmly fixed on the horizon of surveillance. (We worked hard on that analogy!)

Case 3.26: Clot Shot

A 45-year-old man presents to the ED with sudden-onset, sharp epigastric pain that began 24 hours ago. He does not report fevers, nausea, vomiting, or diarrhea. He has no history of liver disease, alcohol use, or recent travel. His past medical history is notable only for treated hypertension. He takes lisinopril but no anticoagulants or hormonal medications.

On exam, he is afebrile with normal vital signs. His abdomen is soft with mild tenderness in the right upper quadrant and epigastrium, but no rebound or guarding. There is no palmar erythema or spider angiomas seen.

Labs show: AST 48 IU/L; ALT 42 IU/L; ALP 91 IU/L; total bilirubin 1.1 mg/dL; INR 1.0; platelet count 380,000/µL.

Abdominal ultrasound with Doppler reveals hypoechoic material within the main portal vein and absent flow on color Doppler. A contrast-enhanced CT confirms acute portal vein thrombosis (PVT) extending into the left and right intrahepatic branches. No signs of cirrhosis or malignancy are noted. He is admitted to the hospital for further management.

Know your guidelines!

1. What are the key steps in evaluating a patient with acute PVT?
2. What hypercoagulable conditions should be considered?
3. When should anticoagulation be started?
4. How is chronic PVT different from acute PVT?
5. What are the potential complications of PVT?

Case 3.26: What do the guidelines say?

Source: ACG 2020 Disorders of Hepatic and Mesenteric Circulation Guideline[186]

Portal vein thrombosis (PVT) often presents in 2 dramatically different ways—a chronic, incidental finding in cirrhosis or a sudden, painful, and potentially dangerous vascular event in someone without liver disease. This case is the latter: a healthy 45-year-old with abdominal pain, no stigmata of chronic liver disease, and imaging that reveals an acute thrombus in the portal vein. The diagnosis is often missed or delayed because the symptoms are nonspecific. But once you spot it, the stakes are high. Prompt recognition and early anticoagulation can prevent bowel infarction, cavernous transformation, or progression to chronic PVT, which can make future interventions—like transplant or portal decompression—much harder.

PVT with vs without cirrhosis are 2 different diseases

The ACG guideline walks us through the evaluation and management of PVT step by step, reminding us that context matters: does the patient have cirrhosis or not? Is this bland thrombus or tumor thrombus? Is it acute or chronic? Each fork leads to a different treatment path (**Figure 3.23**).

Confirming the Diagnosis: Imaging and Anatomy

PVT can be diagnosed on Doppler ultrasound, which can show material within the portal vein and, more definitively, loss of color flow. In this case, as is common, the finding was confirmed on contrast-enhanced CT, which allows for better evaluation of thrombus extent and helps rule out underlying malignancy, particularly HCC, which is the most common cause of tumor thrombus.

When PVT is seen, the next step is to classify it along 3 axes:

1. Acute vs chronic
2. Cirrhotic vs non-cirrhotic
3. Bland (benign) vs malignant (tumor thrombus)

This patient checks the boxes for acute, non-cirrhotic, and bland—

Figure 3.23. *ACG Algorithm for PVT.*[186]

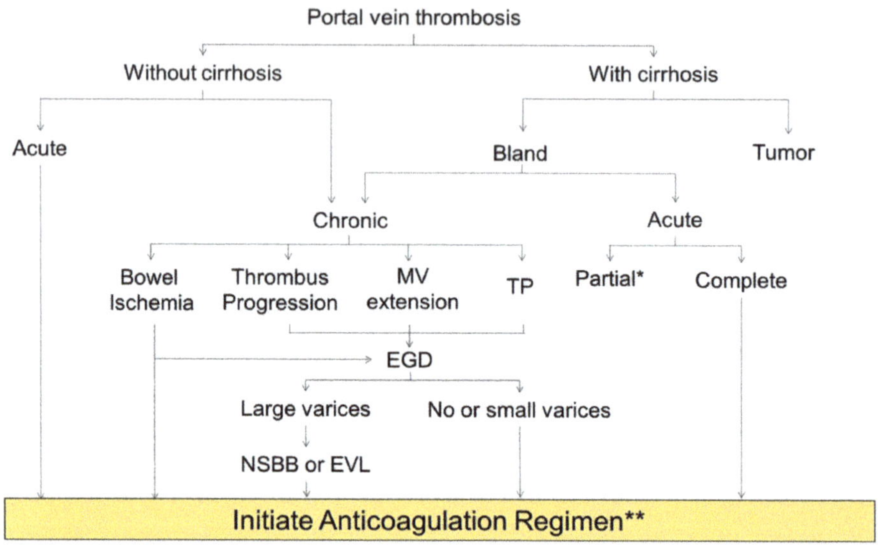

*No anticoagulation except for acute partial thrombosis among liver transplant listed candidates. **Anticoagulation duration: 3-6 months if discrete precipitant and indefinite if thombophilia or patients listed for liver transplantation. EVL, endoscopic variceal ligation; NSBB, nonselective beta-blockers; TP, thombophilia.

the ideal scenario for early and potentially curative anticoagulation. To help frame this discussion, also see **Figure 3.24** for a visual reference of the hepatic and portal venous system anatomy.

Why Did It Happen? Look for the Prothrombotic Clues

In non-cirrhotic patients, PVT is often a red flag for underlying thrombophilia. Thus, testing is recommended for the following conditions with a comprehensive hypercoagulable workup, including:

- Tyrosine kinase janus kinase 2 (JAK2) mutation (to evaluate for a myeloproliferative disorder—the most common thrombophilic etiology of non-cirrhotic PVT)
- Factor V Leiden and prothrombin gene mutations
- Antiphospholipid syndrome
- Protein C, S, and antithrombin deficiencies
- Homocysteine and *MTHFR* mutation (less commonly)

Importantly, some tests (e.g., protein C/S levels) can be misleading

Figure 3.24. *Hepatic and Portal Venous System.*[186]

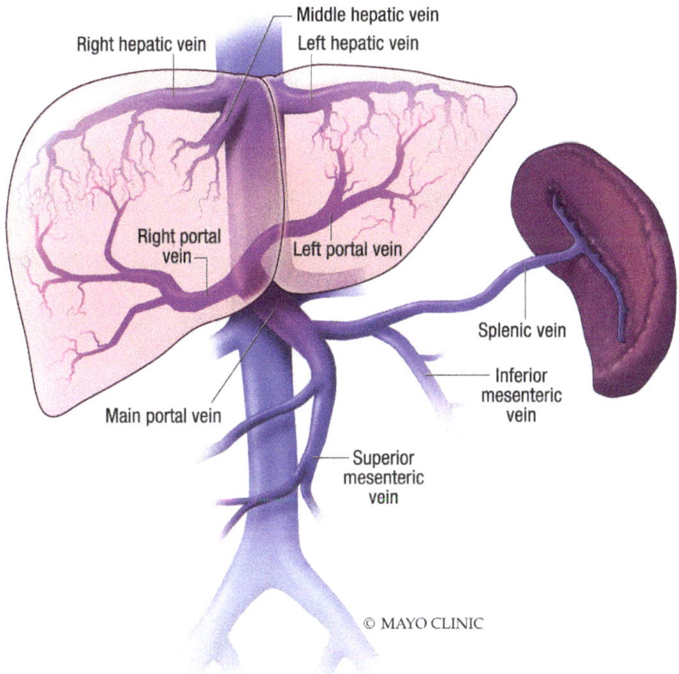

if drawn while the patient is acutely ill or already on anticoagulation, so timing matters.

> Cirrhosis is a prothrombotic state, so thrombophilia testing is not routinely recommended.

In contrast, if this was a patient with cirrhosis, the work-up would be much more limited. Cirrhosis alone alters the coagulation balance and is a recognized prothrombotic state, so thrombophilia testing is not routinely recommended in cirrhosis.

To Treat or Not to Treat? Start the Clock

> Start anticoagulation ASAP when you diagnose PVT without cirrhosis

According to the ACG guideline, anticoagulation should be initiated immediately in all patients with acute PVT without cirrhosis, unless there are contraindications. The goal is complete or partial recanalization and prevention of:

- Thrombus extension into mesenteric veins (which raises the

risk of bowel ischemia)
- Cavernous transformation (collateralization and loss of native portal vein architecture)
- Chronic PVT with variceal complications

Anticoagulation is typically with unfractionated heparin or low molecular weight heparin (LMWH) bridged to warfarin, or increasingly, direct oral anticoagulants (DOACs). By the way, for more on DOACs and GI bleeding, check out *G2G Volume 2.*

Treat PVT for 3-6 months, and indefinitely if there is a persistent hypercoagulable state

Duration of therapy is generally 3-6 months if a reversible cause (e.g., transient prothrombotic trigger, surgery, infection) is found. If the patient is found to have a persistent hypercoagulable condition, indefinite anticoagulation is usually recommended.

Avoiding Pitfalls: Cirrhosis and Varices

In patients with cirrhosis, the decision to anticoagulate is more nuanced. The guideline still supports anticoagulation for acute or progressive PVT, but only after an EGD to assess for esophageal varices. If large varices are found, they must be addressed with non-selective beta-blockers or band ligation prior to initiating therapy. But in non-cirrhotic PVT, as in this case, anticoagulation can proceed without delay.

Chronic PVT: A Different Animal

In chronic, non-progressive PVT in cirrhotics without symptoms, anticoagulation may not not required unless the patient is headed towards liver transplantation

Had this thrombus been chronic—meaning the patient had signs of portal cavernoma, portal hypertension, and no abdominal pain—the approach would be different. In chronic, non-progressive PVT in cirrhotic patients without symptoms, anticoagulation is often not required. However, if the patient is listed for transplantation, anticoagulation is often recommended due to the increased post-transplant mortality with occlusive PVT at the time of transplantation.[188] Nonetheless, in acute cases like this, the guideline is clear: start treatment early to preserve native portal flow.

The Bottom line: This case is a textbook example of acute, non-cirrhotic PVT, a diagnosis that can be easy to miss—but rewarding to catch early. The ACG guideline gives us a clear roadmap: confirm with imaging, rule out cirrhosis and cancer, work up for thrombophilia, and initiate prompt anticoagulation to protect portal flow and prevent long-term complications.

Case 3.27: All Backed Up

A 37-year-old woman presents to the ED with progressive abdominal discomfort and distention, increasing leg swelling, and early satiety. Symptoms have developed gradually over the past 3 weeks. She denies alcohol use or prior liver disease. She has a history of migraines and has been taking a combined oral contraceptive pill (ethinyl estradiol/norgestimate) for 10 years.

On exam, she appears mildly icteric. Vitals are normal. She has shifting dullness, mild RUQ tenderness, and bilateral lower extremity edema. There are no spider angiomas seen. There are no dermatologic stigmata of chronic liver disease.

Labs reveal: ALT 102 IU/L; AST 121 IU/L; ALP 110 IU/L; total bilirubin 2.4 mg/dL; INR 1.4; albumin 3.1 g/dL; platelet count 142,000/µL.

Abdominal ultrasound with Doppler shows hepatomegaly, ascites, and absent flow in the right and middle hepatic veins, with reversal of portal flow.

Know your guidelines!

1. What is the most likely diagnosis?
2. What imaging studies are recommended?
3. What hypercoagulable work-up should be initiated?
4. What is the treatment?
5. What factors determine long-term prognosis and follow-up strategy?

Case 3.27: What do the guidelines say?

Source: ACG 2020 Disorders of Hepatic and Mesenteric Circulation Guideline [186]

Budd-Chiari Syndrome (BCS) is a rare but critical vascular liver disorder caused by hepatic venous outflow obstruction, anywhere from the small hepatic venules up to the inferior vena cava. It's often missed or misattributed to "unexplained ascites" or presumed cirrhosis—especially in young women, where the signs evolve subtly. But BCS has a telltale combination of features: abdominal pain, hepatomegaly, ascites, and hepatic dysfunction, sometimes accompanied by portal hypertension. In our case, a healthy 37-year-old woman develops new-onset ascites, mild jaundice, and elevated liver enzymes—yet no prior liver disease and no clear risk factors. That should always trigger one thought in your mind: Is this Budd-Chiari?

> Think of BCS when there is:
> * Abdominal pain
> * Hepatomegaly
> * Ascites
> * Hepatic dysfunction

Imaging Seals the Diagnosis—Doppler First, CT or MRI for Confirmation

The ACG guideline is clear: Doppler ultrasound is the first-line test, and in this case, it's already pointing in the right direction. The finding of absent flow in the right and middle hepatic veins, hepatomegaly, and reversed portal flow strongly suggest hepatic venous outflow obstruction. But Doppler alone is not always definitive. The next step is a contrast-enhanced CT or MRI, which can demonstrate non-opacified hepatic veins, caudate lobe hypertrophy (a classic board review buzzword phrase! See **Figure 3.25** for an example), and characteristic "flip-flop" enhancement patterns (with delayed central enhancement due to venous congestion). Cross-sectional imaging not only confirms the diagnosis—it helps assess the extent of obstruction and identify patients who may benefit from intervention.

> Caudate lobe hypertrophy should make you think of BCS

If all 3 hepatic veins are thrombosed or compressed, and especially if the caudate lobe is enlarged (due to compensation as blood is

Figure 3.25. *Caudate lobe hypertrophy with homogenous enhancement in BCS.*[189]

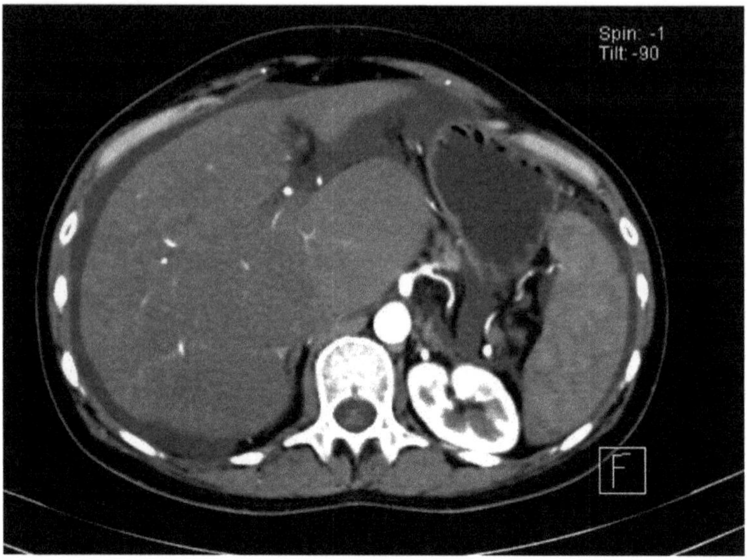

rerouted around the obstructed hepatic venous system to the caudate lobe, since it drains directly into the IVC via the caudate vein), the diagnosis of classic BCS is confirmed.

In uncertain cases, hepatic venography with pressure measurements remains the gold standard. But in most cases, imaging plus clinical context is enough.

Don't Forget the Why: Look for the Underlying Cause

Every patient with BCS warrants a full hypercoagulable work-up, even if the diagnosis seems obvious. There are a lot of potential etiologies and risk factors. The ACG guidelines recommend a hematology consultation for the evaluation and treatment of a specific underlying prothrombotic disorder. At any rate, you should know that about half of BCS cases are due to myeloproliferative neoplasms (MPNs), which are identified by testing for the JAK2 V617F gene mutation in peripheral myeloid cells.[190]

This patient's use of estrogen-containing oral contraceptives is a potential contributor, but estrogen alone rarely causes BCS unless another thrombophilia is present. That's why a "negative work-up" isn't negative until MPNs are excluded.

Stepwise Treatment: Start with Anticoagulation and Escalate from There

1. Start anticoagulation immediately, typically with unfractionated heparin or LMWH transitioning to warfarin or a DOAC (if no contraindication).
2. If symptoms persist (especially ascites or hepatic dysfunction), proceed to angioplasty ± stenting, particularly for segmental or web-like IVC obstruction.
3. If that fails—or if hepatic vein outflow is fully occluded—consider TIPS (transjugular intrahepatic portosystemic shunt) to decompress the liver and improve flow.
4. Liver transplantation is reserved for patients who develop fulminant hepatic failure, progressive hepatic decompensation despite TIPS, or those with HCC.

This "ladder approach" preserves liver function and delays or avoids transplant, and it's crucial to not skip the early steps—most patients respond to anticoagulation or TIPS without needing surgery.

Long-Term Management and Monitoring

Once stabilized, these patients require lifelong anticoagulation, especially if a prothrombotic condition is found. Periodic monitoring includes:

> Once stabilized, BCS requires lifelong anticoagulation if a prothrombotic conditions is found

- Duplex ultrasound to assess hepatic vein flow and detect re-thrombosis or stent dysfunction
- Liver laboratory testing
- Surveillance imaging for HCC in patients with chronic BCS and cirrhosis every 6 months
- Regular follow-up with hepatology and hematology.

This patient, assuming no further decompensation, may be managed with anticoagulation alone—but that hinges on follow-up imaging, symptom monitoring, and collaborative care.

Bringing It Together

Subtle ascites, vague RUQ pain, mild jaundice in a patient without cirrhosis? That's your cue to grab a Doppler. The ACG guidelines give us a clear, tiered strategy: confirm with imaging, search for underlying thrombophilia (especially MPNs), start anticoagulation, and escalate as needed. The key is early recognition and not mistaking a reversible vascular problem for irreversible liver failure. Her liver's not backed up because it's failing—it's failing because it's backed up. Unlock the outflow, and you may just restore the system.

Well, that's a wrap. You've just read the swan song of the G2G trilogy. We hope you enjoyed reading it as much as we enjoyed writing it! It certainly helped us learn a lot and we hope that we were able to pass that on to you.

Liver Quiz

1. A 53-year-old man is referred to hepatology after routine labs show elevated liver enzymes and ferritin. He reports mild fatigue and joint stiffness, but no jaundice or abdominal pain. He does not drink alcohol and has no known liver disease. Labs reveal: Ferritin: 740 ng/mL; Transferrin saturation: 68%; ALT: 58 IU/L; AST: 52 IU/L; Hepatitis B and C panels: negative; Family history: brother with diabetes, father with "liver trouble" What is the most appropriate next step in the evaluation of this patient?

    a. Order a liver biopsy to assess iron burden and stage fibrosis
    b. Refer for phlebotomy to reduce iron overload
    c. Begin iron chelation therapy with deferasirox
    d. Order HFE genetic testing to evaluate for hereditary hemochromatosis
    e. Repeat iron studies in 3-6 months to confirm persistence of abnormal values

2. A 42-year-old man presents with new-onset epigastric pain. He has no history of liver disease. Labs show: AST 48 IU/L; ALT 52 IU/L; total bilirubin 1.0 mg/dL; INR 1.0; platelets 355,000/μL. Doppler ultrasound shows absent flow in the portal vein with hypoechoic material; CT confirms portal vein thrombosis without cirrhosis or malignancy. What is the most appropriate next step?

    a. Refer for transjugular liver biopsy
    b. Start anticoagulation and screen for myeloproliferative neoplasm
    c. Observe without treatment and re-image in 3 months
    d. Begin beta-blocker prophylaxis for varices
    e. Schedule TIPS placement for portal decompression

3. A 35-year-old woman presents with abdominal distension and early satiety. She has been taking oral contraceptives for over a decade. Exam reveals hepatomegaly and ascites. Labs: AST 98 IU/L; ALT 105 IU/L; total bilirubin 2.2 mg/dL; INR 1.3; albumin 2.8 g/dL. Doppler ultrasound shows absent flow in the right and middle hepatic veins. Which of the following is the most appropriate next step?

    a. Begin spironolactone and monitor liver enzymes
    b. Refer for liver transplantation evaluation
    c. Initiate anticoagulation and obtain JAK2 mutation testing
    d. Schedule TIPS placement
    e. Order upper endoscopy to screen for varices

4. A 59-year-old woman with metastatic melanoma on nivolumab presents for routine labs before her next infusion. She feels well. Labs show: ALT 337U/L; AST 320 IU/L; ALP 146 IU/L; total bilirubin 1.0 mg/dL; INR 1.1. She is asymptomatic and not taking any other medications. What is the most appropriate initial management?

   a. Begin prednisone 40 mg daily
   b. Administer intravenous N-acetylcysteine
   c. Perform liver biopsy to confirm diagnosis
   d. Start mycophenolate mofetil and stop immunotherapy permanently
   e. Discontinue nivolumab and monitor liver enzymes closely

5. A 60-year-old man with alcohol-related cirrhosis presents with confusion, drowsiness and fever. Vitals: T 38.8°C; BP 108/64 mmHg; HR 108 bpm. Exam reveals ascites and asterixis. Labs: creatinine 2.6 mg/dL; total bilirubin 6.5 mg/dL; INR 1.8; sodium 130 mmol/L; lactate 3.9 mmol/L. Diagnostic paracentesis shows 520 neutrophils/mm^3. According to the NACSELD definition, how many organ failures does this patient currently have?

   a. 0
   b. 1
   c. 2
   d. 3
   e. 4

6. A 63-year-old man is referred for abnormal liver tests noted during pre-op clearance. He is asymptomatic and reports no alcohol use. Labs: ALP 365 IU/L; ALT 48 IU/L; AST 52 IU/L; total bilirubin 0.9 mg/dL; GGT elevated; ANA and ASMA negative; IgG and IgG4 normal. Right upper quadrant ultrasound shows a normal liver contour, no biliary dilation, and no gallstones. MRCP is also normal. He continues to have an isolated elevation in ALP over several months. Which of the following is the most appropriate next step?

   a. Start a trial of ursodeoxycholic acid
   b. Refer for ERCP
   c. Obtain antimitochondrial antibody
   d. Perform EUS to assess for microlithiasis
   e. Reassure and monitor annually

7. A 44-year-old woman undergoes abdominal CT without contrast for nephrolithiasis, which reveals a 2.7 cm hypodense lesion in the liver. She is asymptomatic, has normal liver enzymes, no history of liver disease, and her AFP is normal. MRI with hepatobiliary contrast shows a homogeneously enhancing lesion in the arterial phase with a central scar and retention of contrast on the hepatobiliary phase. What is the most appropriate next step?

   a. Liver biopsy to rule out hepatocellular carcinoma
   b. Surgical resection due to concern for hepatic adenoma
   c. Repeat MRI in 6 months to confirm stability
   d. No further work-up or follow-up is necessary
   e. Refer for multidisciplinary tumor board evaluation

8. A 59-year-old man with hepatitis C-related cirrhosis (Child-Pugh A) undergoes routine HCC surveillance. Ultrasound detects a 2.1 cm hypoechoic lesion in segment VI. He is asymptomatic. Labs: ALT 54 IU/L; AST 67 IU/L; total bilirubin 1.3 mg/dL; AFP 12 ng/mL. MRI with extracellular contrast shows arterial hyperenhancement and washout on the portal venous phase. The lesion is non-capsulated but well-defined. Which of the following is the best next step?

   a. Repeat MRI in 3 months
   b. Schedule core biopsy of the lesion
   c. Diagnose HCC and refer to a transplant center
   d. Start sorafenib therapy
   e. Obtain PET-CT to rule out extrahepatic disease

9. A 34-year-old woman is found to have a 6.5 cm hepatic lesion on MRI performed for right upper quadrant discomfort. She has no history of liver disease. MRI with hepatobiliary contrast shows arterial phase hyperenhancement and hypointensity on hepatobiliary phase, without a central scar. There is no evidence of washout or hemorrhage. She takes oral contraceptives but is otherwise healthy. Labs are unremarkable. What is the most appropriate next step?

   a. Reassure and repeat imaging in 12 months
   b. Perform percutaneous biopsy to confirm FNH
   c. Stop oral contraceptives and reimage in 6 months
   d. Recommend surgical resection
   e. Initiate empiric anticoagulation

10. A 24-year-old woman presents with nausea and right upper quadrant pain. She admits to taking "many" acetaminophen tablets after a breakup 18 hours ago. On exam, she is awake but mildly confused. Labs: AST 5,800 IU/L; ALT 6,100 IU/L; INR 2.8; total bilirubin 3.2 mg/dL; creatinine 1.6 mg/dL; glucose 58 mg/dL. Which of the following is the most appropriate immediate next step?

    a. Perform urgent liver biopsy
    b. Start intravenous N-acetylcysteine
    c. Initiate corticosteroids for autoimmune hepatitis
    d. Begin empiric broad-spectrum antibiotics
    e. Administer IV vitamin K and observe

11. A 32-year-old woman with no prior liver disease presents with worsening confusion 2 days after an acetaminophen overdose. On exam, she is somnolent and arousable to voice. Labs: INR 6.2; pH 7.15; creatinine 2.1 mg/dL; ALT 4,100 IU/L; AST 3,800 IU/L; total bilirubin 3.6 mg/dL. She is started on IV N-acetylcysteine. According to King's College Criteria, which of the following findings supports an indication for urgent liver transplant referral?

    a. Total bilirubin >3 mg/dL
    b. ALT >2,000 IU/L
    c. Creatinine >1.5 mg/dL
    d. Time to jaundice < 3 days
    e. Arterial pH <7.3

12. A 19-year-old woman presents with jaundice and altered mental status. She has no history of alcohol use or liver disease. Labs: AST 280 IU/L; ALT 130 IU/L; alkaline phosphatase 29 IU/L; total bilirubin 17.6 mg/dL; INR 3.7; creatinine 2.4 mg/dL. Slit lamp exam reveals Kayser-Fleischer rings. Which of the following additional findings would most strongly support a diagnosis of Wilson disease as the cause of her acute liver failure?

    a. Elevated serum ceruloplasmin
    b. AST:ALT ratio <1
    c. Alkaline phosphatase:total bilirubin ratio <2
    d. Serum copper <10 mcg/dL
    e. Macrocytic anemia

13. A 60-year-old woman is referred for elevated ferritin. She feels well and has no liver-related symptoms. Labs: ferritin 980 ng/mL; transferrin saturation 36%; ALT 41 IU/L; AST 39 IU/L. HFE genotyping shows H63D homozygosity. She has a BMI of 32 kg/m^2 and ultrasound shows mild hepatic steatosis without hepatomegaly or nodularity. What is the most appropriate next step?

    a. Begin therapeutic phlebotomy
    b. Order liver biopsy to evaluate for hepatic iron deposition
    c. Reassure; no treatment or further work-up is needed
    d. Counsel on weight loss and monitor liver enzymes and iron studies
    e. Start iron chelation with deferoxamine

14. A 25-year-old woman presents with fatigue and mild right upper quadrant discomfort. Labs show: ALT 314 IU/L; AST 366 IU/L; ALP 104 IU/L; total bilirubin 1.1 mg/dL. ANA is positive at 1:160; smooth muscle antibody titer is 1:40; IgG is mildly elevated. She has been taking minocycline for acne for the past 10 months. Hepatitis serologies are negative. What is the most appropriate next step?

    a. Begin prednisone 40 mg daily for presumed autoimmune hepatitis
    b. Discontinue minocycline and monitor liver tests over 30-60 days
    c. Refer for liver biopsy to confirm diagnosis
    d. Switch to doxycycline and continue treatment
    e. Repeat autoimmune panel and IgG in 6 weeks

15. A 66-year-old man presents with jaundice and pruritus 2 weeks after completing a 10-day course of amoxicillin-clavulanate for sinusitis. He denies abdominal pain, fever, or alcohol use. Labs: ALP 418 IU/L; ALT 88 IU/L; AST 76 IU/L; total bilirubin 5.1mg/dL; GGT elevated; INR 1.1. Hepatitis serologies are negative; ultrasound shows no biliary dilation or stones. Which of the following is the most appropriate next step?

    a. Start prednisone 40 mg daily
    b. Refer for ERCP
    c. Monitor liver tests and provide symptomatic treatment
    d. Order MRCP to evaluate for PSC
    e. Perform liver biopsy to guide management

16. A 62-year-old woman with NASH cirrhosis presents with fatigue and low urine output after several days of vomiting and poor oral intake. She is taking furosemide and spironolactone. On exam, she is volume depleted and oriented. Labs: creatinine 2.5 mg/dL (baseline 0.9); sodium 129 mmol/L; total bilirubin 3.4 mg/dL; INR 1.4; urine microscopy is bland. After 2 days of IV albumin and stopping diuretics, creatinine remains 2.7 mg/dL. Which of the following best supports a diagnosis of hepatorenal syndrome acute kidney injury?

    a. Hyaline casts on urine microscopy
    b. Proteinuria >500 mg/day
    c. Lack of improvement after IVF resuscitation
    d. Response to midodrine and octreotide
    e. Elevated BUN:creatinine ratio

17. A 54-year-old man with alcohol-related cirrhosis is admitted with sepsis from pneumonia. He develops grade 3 hepatic encephalopathy, creatinine 3.2 mg/dL, INR 2.2, and requires norepinephrine for hypotension. He is intubated for airway protection. Total bilirubin is 12.6 mg/dL. The ICU team diagnoses ACLF-3. His blood pressure improves and oxygen requirement decreases the next day. What is the most appropriate approach regarding liver transplantation?

    a. Delay transplant referral until infection is fully resolved
    b. Proceed with transplant referral
    c. Decline transplant as ACLF-3 is an absolute contraindication
    d. Wait for bilirubin and INR to stabilize before evaluating
    e. Refer only if the patient remains intubated >7 days

18. A 58-year-old man with hepatitis B cirrhosis is admitted with lethargy, abdominal pain, and fever. Vitals: BP 102/62 mmHg; HR 110 bpm; T 38.7°C. Labs: creatinine 2.3 mg/dL; INR 1.5; bilirubin 7.8 mg/dL. Exam reveals grade 3 hepatic encephalopathy. He requires 4 L of oxygen by nasal cannula for an SpO_2 of 92%. Chest x-ray shows right lower lobe pneumonia. Based on NACSELD criteria, how many organ failures does he currently have?

    a. 1
    b. 2
    c. 3
    d. 4
    e. Cannot be determined without MELD score

19. A 67-year-old woman is referred for evaluation of isolated alkaline phosphatase elevation. Labs: ALP 416 IU/L; ALT 28 IU/L; AST 29 IU/L; total bilirubin 0.7 mg/dL; GGT is elevated. AMA is negative. Ultrasound and MRCP are unremarkable. She is asymptomatic. Which of the following diagnoses is least likely to be responsible for this biochemical profile?

    a. IgG4-related cholangitis
    b. Small duct primary sclerosing cholangitis
    c. Hepatic lymphoma
    d. Autoimmune hepatitis
    e. Primary biliary cholangitis

20. A 28-year-old man is brought to the ED with confusion, jaundice, and nausea. He takes no medications and there is no known history of drug or alcohol use. Labs: AST 3,600 IU/L; ALT 3,400 IU/L; ALP 112 IU/L; total bilirubin 4.8 mg/dL; INR 2.1. CT abdomen is unremarkable; hepatitis serologies and acetaminophen level are pending. Which of the following would be least likely to cause this pattern of liver injury?

    a. Acute Budd-Chiari syndrome
    b. Autoimmune hepatitis
    c. Acute viral hepatitis
    d. Alcohol-associated hepatitis
    e. Ischemic hepatitis

21. A 62-year-old man with hepatitis C cirrhosis undergoes surveillance ultrasound, which detects a 1.5 cm hypoechoic lesion in segment VII. AFP is 8 ng/mL. MRI with contrast shows arterial phase hyperenhancement without washout. There is no capsule or fat. What is the most appropriate next step?
    a. Diagnose HCC and refer for transplant
    b. Perform liver biopsy of the lesion
    c. Begin sorafenib therapy
    d. Monitor with ultrasound every 6 months
    e. Repeat MRI or CT in 3 months

22. A 72-year-old man is admitted for evaluation of worsening jaundice and confusion. Labs: ALT 68 IU/L; AST 74 IU/L; ALP 120 IU/L; total bilirubin 6.2 mg/dL; albumin 2.4 g/dL; INR 2.3. The intern states, "His LFTs are only mildly elevated." Which of the following best reflects the true liver function tests?

    a. ALT, AST, and ALP
    b. ALT, AST, and total bilirubin
    c. Albumin, INR, and total bilirubin
    d. Albumin and alkaline phosphatase
    e. GGT, INR, and ALT

23. A 30-year-old woman presents with fatigue and abnormal liver tests discovered on routine labs. She has been taking minocycline for acne for the past 6 months. Labs: ALT 970 IU/L; AST 820 IU/L; ALP 108 IU/L; total bilirubin 1.1 mg/dL. ANA is positive at 1:320; IgG is mildly elevated. She denies alcohol or herbal supplement use. What is the best description of this patient's pattern of liver injury?
    a. Hepatocellular
    b. Cholestatic
    c. Mixed
    d. Ischemic
    e. Tumor-related

24. 78-year-old man with compensated cirrhosis due to hepatitis B is found to have non-occlusive chronic portal vein thrombosis on surveillance imaging. He has no history of GI bleeding, and his only medication is tenofovir. He is asymptomatic, with preserved liver function and no evidence of bowel ischemia with small esophageal varices on recent EGD without stigmata. Which of the following is the most appropriate next step?

    a. Begin indefinite anticoagulation
    b. Refer for TIPS placement
    c. Order thrombophilia panel
    d. Start non-selective beta-blocker and observe
    e. Refer for transplant evaluation

25. A 64-year-old woman with a history of breast cancer in remission is found to have a new 3.1 cm liver lesion on abdominal CT done for nonspecific abdominal pain. She has no liver disease. MRI with extracellular contrast shows a hypovascular lesion without arterial enhancement or washout. The lesion is not clearly cystic or classic for hemangioma or FNH. What is the most appropriate next step?

    a. Reassure and repeat imaging in 6 months
    b. Schedule percutaneous biopsy
    c. Refer for surgical resection
    d. Start empiric chemotherapy
    e. Diagnose hepatic adenoma and observe

26. A 56-year-old man with alcohol-related cirrhosis presents with lethargy and abdominal discomfort. Vitals: T 38.5°C; BP 102/64 mmHg; HR 104 bpm. Exam reveals shifting dullness and mild encephalopathy. Labs: WBC 12,000/μL; creatinine 1.8 mg/dL; total bilirubin 4.1 mg/dL. Paracentesis reveals 320 neutrophils/mm^3; ascitic protein 1.0 g/dL; culture is pending. What is the most appropriate initial management?

    a. Observe and repeat paracentesis in 48 hours
    b. Start empiric antibiotics and IV albumin
    c. Begin rifaximin and lactulose
    d. Wait for culture results before starting antibiotics
    e. Refer for TIPS placement

27. A 59-year-old man presents with nausea, lethargy, and jaundice. He has a history of heavy alcohol use but no known liver disease. Labs: AST 2,800 IU/L; ALT 1,300 IU/L; ALP 98 IU/L; total bilirubin 1.7 mg/dL; INR 2.4. He is somnolent but arousable. Acetaminophen level is undetectable. Hepatitis serologies are pending. Which of the following best explains why alcohol is unlikely to be the sole cause of this patient's transaminase elevation?

    a. AST is greater than ALT
    b. ALP is relatively normal
    c. The AST:ALT ratio is >2
    d. The magnitude of AST and ALT elevation exceeds typical alcohol-associated hepatitis
    e. The bilirubin is >5 mg/dL

28. For the patient above, which of the following would be the most appropriate to order to determine a potentially treatable cause of the acute liver test abnormalities?

    a. Serum ceruloplasmin
    b. Antimitochondrial antibody (AMA)
    c. Herpes simplex virus (HSV) PCR
    d. Iron panel and HFE genotyping
    e. Alpha-1 antitrypsin phenotype

29. A 31-year-old woman presents with fever, abdominal pain, and malaise. She is 22 weeks pregnant and has no history of liver disease. Exam reveals right upper quadrant tenderness without rash or mucosal lesions. Labs: AST 2,300 IU/L; ALT 2,600 IU/L; ALP 102 IU/L; total bilirubin 1.9 mg/dL; INR 2.6; creatinine 1.8 mg/dL; ANA and SMA are normal. Hepatitis A, B, and C serologies and serum toxicology screen including acetaminophen level are all negative. What is the most appropriate next step?

    a. Begin IV acyclovir
    b. Perform liver biopsy
    c. Start prednisone for presumed autoimmune hepatitis
    d. Wait for HSV PCR before initiating therapy
    e. Recommend immediate delivery

30. A 38-year-old man with no past medical history presents with jaundice and confusion after 4 days of nausea and malaise. He denies medication use, alcohol, or toxin exposure. On exam, he is disoriented to time and place. Labs: ALT 2,800 IU/L; AST 3,100 IU/L; INR 5.1; total bilirubin 8.6 mg/dL; arterial pH 7.38; creatinine 2.7 mg/dL. Hepatitis A IgM is positive. What is the most appropriate next step?

    a. Begin corticosteroids for fulminant autoimmune hepatitis
    b. Observe and repeat labs in 12-24 hours
    c. Start empiric acyclovir
    d. Refer for urgent liver transplant evaluation
    e. Repeat arterial blood gas to assess for metabolic acidosis

31. A 35-year-old man presents with anxiety and fatigue to the urgent care clinic. He admits to drinking gin to help with his anxiety. His BMI is 24 and his labs show AST 102 IU/L, ALT 52 IU/L, total bilirubin 0.8 mg/dL, albumin 4.2 g/dL, INR 1.0. Ultrasound is consistent with fatty liver and no masses seen. Besides abstinence, what should you recommend?

    a. Liver biopsy
    b. Prednisolone
    c. Cognitive behavioral therapy
    d. MRI of the liver
    e. Weight loss with diet and exercise

32. A 67-year-old man with ALD has been unable to stop drinking alcohol despite knowing the harmful risks. He is seen in the emergency department after a fall, after slipping on the stairs at home. His foot X-ray shows no fracture, and he is diagnosed with an ankle sprain. He is given a protective boot and ankle wrap. He does mention that he has noticed generalized muscle mass loss over the past few months but does not want any further evaluation or testing. Which of the options below is the best choice?

    a. Admit him to inpatient alcohol rehabilitation
    b. Call security services so he can be held against his will so you can provide further evaluation and treatment
    c. Call his children to explain the current situation to them so they can help
    d. Advise him to have a late night snack daily
    e. Prescribe prednisolone 40 mg x 28 days

33. A 41-year-old woman with AUD and obesity presents with progressive fatigue, jaundice and muscle wasting. She notes increased alcohol consumption and smoking cigarettes after gastric bypass surgery. She vows never to smoke or drink again. Which of the following is not a risk factor for the progression of ALD?

    a. Obesity
    b. Smoking
    c. Gender
    d. Gastric bypass surgery
    e. High protein diet

34. A 54-year-old man is admitted with severe AH with MELD = 29 and creatinine 1.3. He mentions that he was diagnosed with a "stomach ulcer" when he was young and had "belly pains." He denies any GI bleeding signs or symptoms. He has a history of chronic HBV and has not complied with follow-up or therapy as recommended. He also has diabetes with hemoglobin A1c = 6.1%. To reduce his short-term mortality risk, prednisolone therapy has been contemplated. Which of the following is a contraindication to commencing corticosteroids?

   a. His current MELD score
   b. His abnormal creatinine
   c. Diabetes under control
   d. Untreated chronic HBV
   e. History of peptic ulcer disease

35. A 45-year-old woman is admitted with severe AH with MELD = 32 after a recent binge after a divorce. Ultrasound shows no biliary obstruction. She is started on prednisolone and NAC. After 5 days, her total bilirubin has increased even further. She vows to never drink again and is surrounded by supportive family members, whom she had planned to live with. What is the most appropriate next step?

   a. Cross-sectional liver imaging
   b. Palliative care consult
   c. Referral for early liver transplant evaluation
   d. Add pentoxifylline
   e. Add amoxicillin/clavulanate

36. A 33-year-old primigravid woman presents to your office for consultation at 35 weeks' gestation due to concern for gastrointestinal or liver disease. She describes early satiety without vomiting or weight loss. There has been no jaundice, fever, abdominal pain or change in bowel habits. She is noted to have palmar erythema. ALT 23 IU/L, AST 21 IU/L, ALP 230 IU/L, albumin 3.3 g/dL, total bilirubin 0.8 mg/dL. Which of the following is considered abnormal for this clinical scenario?

   a. Elevated alkaline phosphatase
   b. Low albumin
   c. Early satiety
   d. Palmar erythema
   e. None of the above

37. Which of the following liver diseases unique to pregnancy has a generally normal histological appearance on liver biopsy?

   a. Intrahepatic cholestasis of pregnancy
   b. Acute fatty liver disease of pregnancy
   c. Hyperemesis gravidarum
   d. Eclampisa, preeclampsia
   e. HELLP syndrome

38. Which of the following liver diseases unique to pregnancy is associated with rapid hepatic deterioration often with encephalopathy, hypoglycemia, coagulopathy, hyperbilirubinemia, and marked elevations in aminotransferases?

   a. Intrahepatic cholestasis of pregnancy
   b. Acute fatty liver disease of pregnancy
   c. Hyperemesis gravidarum
   d. Eclampsia/preeclampsia
   e. HELLP syndrome

39. An 81-year-old man was admitted with jaundice and ascites after a recent alcohol binge. He has a long history of alcohol misuse and does not seek regular primary care. He had paracentesis, which showed no evidence of SBP. Unfortunately, he did not respond to corticosteroids and had progression of hyperbilirubinemia and encephalopathy. He is now in the ICU on mechanical ventilation due to aspiration pneumonia with a high oxygen requirement. Which of the following is the most appropriate next step?

   a. Pentoxifylline salvage therapy
   b. Retrial of prednisolone with NAC
   c. Urgent referral for liver transplant evaluation
   d. Palliative care consultation
   e. Empiric intravenous antifungal therapy

40. A 32-year-old man is seen in the ED for a fractured wrist after a recent fall. You review his previous records and find that he has had multiple ED encounters for similar accidents and also for anxiety. You suspect hazardous drinking. Which of the following questions is not part of the AUDIT-C Test that can help identify patients who may have an alcohol use disorder?

a. How often do others feel guilt for your drinking?
b. How often do you have a drink containing alcohol?
c. How many drinks do you have on a typical day when you are drinking?
d. How often do you have 6 or more drinks on 1 occasion?

Answers to Liver Guidelines Quiz

1.	D	21.	E
2.	B	22.	C
3.	C	23.	A
4.	E	24.	D
5.	B	25.	B
6.	C	26.	B
7.	D	27.	D
8.	C	28.	C
9.	D	29.	A
10.	B	30.	D
11.	E	31.	C
12.	C	32.	D
13.	D	33.	E
14.	B	34.	D
15.	C	35.	C
16.	C	36.	E
17.	B	37.	C
18.	A	38.	B
19.	D	39.	D
20.	D	40.	A

ACKNOWLEDGEMENTS

We sincerely thank the authors of the ACG guidelines covered in this book who provided expert review on their sections: Jasmohan Bajaj, MD, MS, FACG; Naga Chalasani, MD, FACG; B. Joseph Elmunzer, MD, MSc; Carrie Frenette, MD; Timothy Gardner, MD, MS, FACG; Patrick Kamath, MD; Kris Kowdley, MD, FACG; Paul Kwo, MD, FACG; Linda Lee, MD, FACG, Keith D. Lindor, MD; Craig McClain, MD, FACG; Alexandra Shingina, MD, MSc; Ashwani Singal, MD, FACG; Tram Tran, MD, FACG; and Santhi Swaroop Vege, MD, MACG. We are grateful to Anjana Pillai, MD, FACG and Romil Saxena, MD for providing original images. In addition, we thank Executive Director Brad Stillman, Director of Scholarly Publications and Managing Editor Claire Neumann, and the ACG Board of Trustees for supporting this successful venture. Special thanks also to the entire ACG staff, who helped along the way, including Neen LeMaster, Angélica Bermúdez, and Liz Starnes. We appreciate feedback from our growing readership for supporting our educational goals.

Personal Dedications

H.K.: To my father, Arvind – for always believing in me, and for giving me the confidence and freedom to chase my dreams as long as I can remember. *Iamque opus exegi*. Om Shanti Shanti Shanti.

B.S.: To my children, Kaelen and Shane, just for being who they are. I love you both deeply.

MEET THE AUTHORS

Brennan Spiegel, MD, MSHS, FACG

Dr. Spiegel is the Dorothy and George Gourrich Chair in Digital Health Ethics at Cedars-Sinai, Founding Director of the Cedars-Sinai Master's Program in Health Delivery Science, and an ACG Governor for Southern California. He is the immediate past Editor-in-Chief for *The American Journal of Gastroenterology* and inaugural Editor-in-Chief for the *Journal of Medical Extended Reality*. Dr. Spiegel has published widely in the fields of health services research, digital health, use of virtual reality in medicine, and clinical gastroenterology across a range of topics. Together with Dr. Karsan, he also wrote the "Acing the GI Board Exam" series of books.

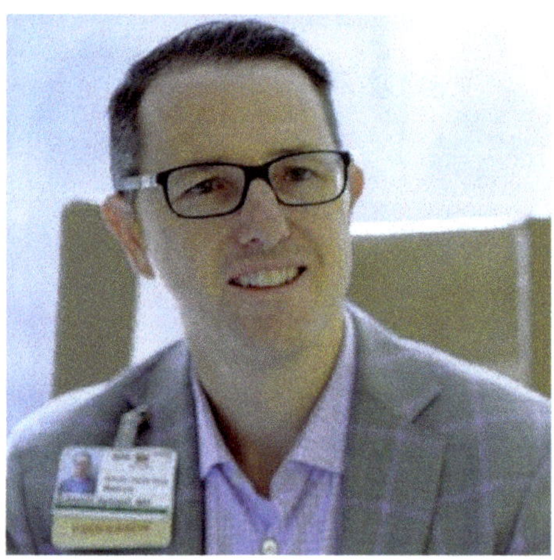

Hetal A. Karsan, MD, FACG

Dr. Karsan is the Chair of Medical Education for United Digestive and Adjunct Professor of Medicine in the Division of Digestive Diseases at Emory University. He serves as the Chair of the Credentials Committee, International Governor, and Governor of Georgia for the ACG. He is the immediate past Editor of the Red Section and Associate Editor for *The American Journal of Gastroenterology*. He has practiced for more than 20 years in both private and academic settings, while actively maintaining board certifications in Gastroenterology, Transplant Hepatology and Internal Medicine. Collaborating with Dr. Spiegel, he wrote the "Acing the GI Board Exam" series of textbooks.

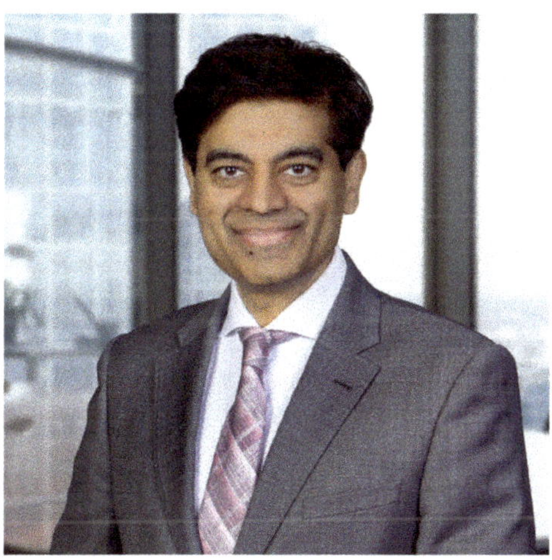

Authors' Note

We wrote this book using good old-fashioned human intelligence. After writing the text, we employed a combination of Chat GPT-4o and o3 to help copyedit the passages. We believe it remains important that humans—not computers—write for other humans, but also recognize benefits of AI to support editing of original text written by humans.

Guidelines covered in *The Guide to the Guidelines* Series

VOLUME 1

- Diagnosis and Management of Eosinophilic Esophagitis (2013)
- Genetic Testing and Management of Hereditary Gastrointestinal Cancer Syndromes (2015)
- Colonoscopy Quality Indicators (2015)
- Management of Dyspepsia (2017)
- Small Intestinal Bacterial Overgrowth (2020)
- Diagnosis and Management of Achalasia (2020)
- Colorectal Cancer Screening (2021)
- Management of Irritable Bowel Syndrome (2021)
- Management of Benign Anorectal Disorders (2021)
- Diagnosis and Management of Gastroesophageal Reflux Disease (2021)
- Gastroparesis (2022)
- Diagnosis and Management of Barrett's Esophagus (2022)
- Pharmacological Management of Chronic Idiopathic Constipation (2023)
- Diagnosis and Management of Gastrointestinal Subepithelial Lesions (2023)

- USMSTF Recommendations: Optimizing Adequacy of Bowel Cleansing for Colonoscopy (2014)
- USMSTF Guidelines on Genetic Evaluation and Management of Lynch Syndrome (2014)
- USMSTF Recommendations: Colonoscopy Surveillance after Colorectal Cancer Resection (2016)
- USMSTF Consensus Statement: Fecal Immunochemical Testing to Screen for Colorectal Neoplasia (2017)
- USMSTF Consensus Statement: Follow-Up After Colonoscopy and Polypectomy (2020)
- USMSTF Recommendations: Endoscopic Removal of Colorectal Lesions (2020)
- USMSTF Recommendations: Endoscopic Recognition and Management Strategies for Malignant Colorectal Polyps (2020)

Volume 2

- Epidemiology, Risk Factors, Patterns of Presentation, Diagnosis, and Management of Colon Ischemia (2015)
- Diagnosis, Treatment and Prevention of Acute Diarrheal Infections in Adults (2016)
- Management of Crohn's Disease in Adults (2018)
- Ulcerative Colitis in Adults (2019)
- Prevention, Diagnosis, and Treatment of *Clostridioides difficile* Infections (2021)
- Upper Gastrointestinal and Ulcer Bleeding (2021)
- Management of Anticoagulants and Antiplatelets During Acute Gastrointestinal Bleeding and the Periendoscopic Period (2022)
- Management of Patients With Acute Lower Gastrointestinal Bleeding (2023)
- Diagnosis and Management of Celiac Disease (2023)
- Treatment of *Helicobacter pylori* Infection (2024)

Volume 3

- Primary Sclerosing Cholangitis (2015)
- Pregnancy and Liver Diseases (2016)
- Evaluation of Abnormal Liver Chemistries (2017)
- Diagnosis and Management of Pancreatic Cysts (2018)
- Hereditary Hemochromatosis (2019)
- Chronic Pancreatitis (2020)
- Disorders of the Hepatic and Mesenteric Circulation (2020)
- Diagnosis and Management of Idiosyncratic Drug-Induced Liver Injury (2021)
- Acute-on-Chronic Liver Failure (2022)
- Acute Liver Failure (2023)
- Diagnosis and Management of Biliary Strictures (2023)
- Management of Acute Pancreatitis (2024)
- Alcohol-Associated Liver Disease (2024)
- Focal Liver Lesions (2024)
- Malnutrition and Nutritional Recommendations in Liver

REFERENCES

1. Tenner S, Vege SS, Sheth SG, et al. American College of Gastroenterology Guidelines: Management of Acute Pancreatitis. Am J Gastroenterol. 2024.119(3):419-437

2. Reisman A, Cho HJ, Holzer H. Unnecessary repeat enzyme testing in acute pancreatitis: A teachable moment. JAMA Intern Med. 2018;178(5):702–3.

3. Semler MW, Self WH, Wanderer JP, et al. Balanced crystalloids versus saline in critically ill adults. N Engl J Med. 2018;378(9):829–839.

4. Signoretti M, Baccini F, Piciucchi M, et al. Repeated transabdominal ultrasonography is a simple and accurate strategy to diagnose a biliary etiology of acute pancreatitis. Pancreas. 2014;43(7):1106–1110.

5. Yadav D, O'Connell M, Papachristou GI. Natural history following the first attack of acute pancreatitis. Am J Gastroenterol. 2012;107(7):1096–1103.

6. Umans DS, Rangkuti CK, Sperna Weiland CJ, et al. Endoscopic ultrasonography can detect a cause in the majority of patients with idiopathic acute pancreatitis: A systematic review and meta-analysis. Endoscopy. 2020;52(11):955–964.

7. Wan J, Ouyang Y, Yu C, et al. Comparison of EUS with MRCP in idiopathic acute pancreatitis: A systematic review and meta-analysis. Gastrointest Endosc. 2018;87(5):1180–8.e9.

8. Wu BU, Johannes RS, Sun X, et al. The early prediction of mortality in acute pancreatitis: A large population-based study. Gut. 2008;57(12): 1698–1703.

9. Forsmark CE, Vege SS, Wilcox CM. Acute pancreatitis. N Engl J Med. 2016;375(20):1972–1981.

10. Yao Q, Liu P, Peng S, et al. Effects of immediate or early oral feeding on acute pancreatitis: A systematic review and meta-analysis. Pancreatology. 2022;22(2):175–184.

11. Singh N, Sharma B, Sharma M, et al. Evaluation of early enteral feeding through nasogastric and nasojejunal tube in severe acute pancreatitis: A noninferiority randomized controlled trial. Pancreas. 2012;41(1):153–159.

12. UK Working Party on Acute Pancreatitis. UK guidelines for the management of acute pancreatitis. Gut. 2005;54(Suppl 3):iii1–9.

13. Tenner S, Baillie J, DeWitt J, et al; American College of Gastroenterology guideline: Management of acute pancreatitis. Am J Gastroenterol. 2013;108(9):1400–15; 1416.

14. Saleh H, Nimma IR, Huang Y, et al. A rare case of sigmoid colon perforation in a patient with severe acute pancreatitis. ACG Case Rep J. 2024;11(5):e01357.

15. Zaheer A, Singh VK, Qureshi RO, et al. The revised Atlanta classification for acute pancreatitis: Updates in imaging terminology and guidelines. Abdom Imaging. 2012;38(1):125–136.

16. Sandhu S, Alhankawi D, Chintanaboina, J, et al. Abstract S1496: Emphysematous pancreatitis mimicking bowel perforation. Am J Gastroenterol. 115:S754-S755.

17. Isenmann R, Runzi M, Kron M, et al. Prophylactic antibiotic treatment in patients with predicted severe acute pancreatitis: A placebo-controlled, double-blind trial. Gastroenterology. 2004;126(4):997–1004.

18. Bakker OJ, van Santvoort HC, van Brunschot S, et al. Endoscopic transgastric vs surgical necrosectomy for infected necrotizing pancreatitis; a randomized trial. JAMA. 2012;307(10):1053–1061.

19. ASGE Standards of Practice Committee; Buxbaum JL, Abbas Fehmi SM, Sultan S, et al. ASGE guideline on the role of endoscopy in the evaluation and management of choledocholithiasis. Gastrointest Endosc. 2019 Jun;89(6):1075-1105.

20. Acosta JM, Ledesma CL. Gallstone migration as a cause of acute pancreatitis. N Engl J Med. 1974;290(9):484–487.

21. Da Costa DW, Dijksman LM, Bouwense SA, et al. Cost-effectiveness of same-admission versus interval cholecystectomy after mild gallstone pancreatitis in the PONCHO trial. Br J Surg. 2016;103(12):1695–1703.

22. Buxbaum JL, Freeman M, Amateau SK, et al. American Society for Gastrointestinal Endoscopy Guideline on post-ERCP pancreatitis prevention strategies: Summary and recommendations. Gastrointest Endosc. 2023;97(2):153–162.

23. Umans DS, Hallensleben ND, Verdonk RC, et al. Recurrence of idiopathic acute pancreatitis after cholecystectomy: Systematic review and meta-analysis. Br J Surg. 2020;107(3):191–199.

24. Cotton PB, Pauls Q, Keith J, et al. Effect of endoscopic sphincterotomy for suspected sphincter of Oddi dysfunction on pain-related disability following cholecystectomy: The EPISOD randomized clinical trial. JAMA. 2014;311(20):2101–2109.

25. Gardner TB, Adler DG, Forsmark CE, Sauer BG, Taylor JR, Whitcomb DC. ACG Clinical Guideline: Chronic pancreatitis. Am J Gastroenterol. 2020;115:322-339.

26. Gardner TB, Levy MJ. EUS diagnosis of chronic pancreatitis. Gastrointest Endosc. 2010;71(7):1280–1289.

27. Madzak A, Olesen SS, Wathle GK, et al. Secretin-stimulated magnetic resonance imaging assessment of the benign pancreatic disorders: Systematic review and proposal for a standardized protocol. Pancreas. 2016;45(8):1092–1103.

28. Iglesias-García J, Lariño-Noia J, Lindkvist B, et al. Endoscopic ultrasound in the diagnosis of chronic pancreatitis. Rev Esp Enferm Dig. 2015 Apr;107(4):221-8.

29. Catalano MF, Sahai A, Levy M, et al. EUS-based criteria for the diagnosis of chronic pancreatitis: The Rosemont classification. Gastrointest Endosc. 2009;69:1251–1261

30. Jha P. Chronic pancreatitis - chain of lakes. Case study, Radiopaedia.org. Accessed 13 Jul 2025. https://doi.org/10.53347/rID-16287.

31. Bhardwaj P, Garg PK, Maulik SK, et al. A randomized controlled trial of antioxidant supplementation for pain relief in patients with chronic pancreatitis. Gastroenterology. 2009;136(1):149–159.

32. Park W, Manickavasagan H, Kumar A. Efficacy of celiac plexus block in chronic pancreatitis: A systematic review. Gastrointest Endo. 2017: AB341–AB342.

33. Chinnakotla S, Beilman GJ, Dunn TB, et al. Factors predicting outcomes after a total pancreatectomy and islet autotransplantation lessons learned from over 500 cases. Ann Surg. 2015;262:610–622.

34. Ranschaert E. Autoimmune pancreatitis. Case study, Radiopaedia.org. Accessed 13 Jul 2025. https://doi.org/10.53347/rID-11060.

35. Elta, GH, Enestvedt BK, Sauer BG, Lennon AM. ACG Clinical Guideline: Diagnosis and management of pancreatic cysts. Am J Gastroenterol. 2018;113(4);464-479.

36. Oh HC, Kim MH, Hwang CY, et al. Cystic lesions of the pancreas: Challenging issues in clinical practice. Am J Gastroenterol. 2008;103(1):229-39.

37. Malekzadeh S, Cannella R, Fournier I, et al. The diagnostic value of abbreviated MRI protocol in the surveillance of Branch-Duct intraductal papillary mucinous neoplasm. Eur J Radiol. 2024:175:111455.

38. Vege SS, Ziring B, Jain R, et al. American Gastroenterological Association Institute guideline on the diagnosis and management of asymptomatic neoplastic pancreatic cysts. Gastroenterology. 2015;148:819–822.

39. Elmunzer BJ, Maranki JL, Gomez V, et al. ACG Clinical Guideline: Diagnosis and management of biliary strictures. Am J Gastroenterol. 2023;118:405-426.

40. de Moura DTH, Ryou M, de Moura EGH, et al. Endoscopic ultrasound-guided fine needle aspiration and endoscopic retrograde cholangiopancreatography-based tissue sampling in suspected malignant biliary strictures: A meta-analysis of same-session procedures. Clin Endosc. 2020;53(4):417–428.

41. van der Gaag NA, Rauws EAJ, van Eijck CHJ, et al. Preoperative biliary drainage for cancer of the head of the pancreas. N Engl J Med. 2010;362(2):129–137.

42. Burnett AS, Calvert TJ, Chokshi RJ. Sensitivity of endoscopic retrograde cholangiopancreatography standard cytology: 10-y review of the literature. J Surg Res. 2013;184(1):304–311.

43. Angsuwatcharakon P, Kulpatcharapong S, Moon JH, et al. Consensus guidelines on the role of cholangioscopy to diagnose intermediate biliary stricture. HPB (Oxford). 2022;24(1):17-29.

44. Zoundjiekpon VD, Falt P, Zapleta J, et al. Fluorescence in situ hybridization in primary diagnosis of biliary strictures: A single-center prospective interventional study. Biomedicines. 2023;11(3):755 1-12.

45. Aggarwal M, Simadibrata DM, Kipp BR, et al. Diagnostic accuracy performance of fluorescence in situ hybridization (FISH) for biliary strictures: A systematic review and meta-analysis. Clin Med. 2024 Oct 28;13(21):6457.

46. Kamal F, Ali Khan M, Lee-Smith W, Sharma S, et al. Metal versus plastic stents in the management of benign biliary strictures: systemic review and meta-analysis of randomized controlled trials. Eur J Gastroenterol Hepatol. 2022 May 1;34(5):478-487.

47. Coté GA, Slivka A, Tarnasky P, et al. Effect of covered metallic stents compared with plastic stents on benign biliary stricture resolution: A randomized clinical trial. JAMA. 2016;315(12):1250–1257.

48. Ramchandani M, Lakhtakia S, Costamagna G, et al. Fully covered self expanding metal stent vs multiple plastic stents to treat benign biliary strictures secondary to chronic pancreatitis: A multicenter randomized trial. Gastroenterology. 2021;161(1):185–195.

49. Karwa S, Patil VV. Role of magnetic resonance cholangiopancreatography in biliary disorders. Int J Radiol Radiat Ther. 2017;2(4):95-99.

50. Gerhards MF, Vos P, van Gulik TM, Rauws EA, Bosma A, Gouma DJ. Incidence of benign lesions in patients resected for suspicious hilar obstruction. Br J Surg. 2001;88:48–51.

51. Verbeek PC, van Leeuwen DJ, de Wit LT, Reeders JW, Simits NJ, Bosma A, et al. Benign fibrosing disease at the hepatic confluence mimicking Klatskin tumors. Surgery. 1992;112:866–871.

52. Heimbach JK, Sanchez W, Rosen CB, et al. Trans-peritoneal fine needle aspiration biopsy of hilar cholangiocarcinoma is associated with disease dissemination. HPB. 2011;13:356–360.

53. Dumonceau J-M, Tringali A, Papanikolaou IS, et al. Endoscopic biliary stenting: Indications, choice of stents, and results: European Society of Gastrointestinal Endoscopy (ESGE) clinical guideline: Updated October 2017. Endoscopy. 2018;50(9):910–30.

54. Castaño Llano Rodrigo. Tumor de la confluencia hiliar hepática (Klatskin). Rev Col Gastroenterol. 2011;26(2):121-30.

55. Ikezawa K, Takada R, Takahashi H, et al. Efficacy of larger-diameter plastic stent placement for preoperative biliary drainage in patients receiving neoadjuvant chemoradiation for pancreatic cancer. Pancreas. 2020; 49(3):e20-e21.

56. Sundaram S, Kiran S, Mazumdar S, et al. Overlap syndrome between primary biliary cholangitis and primary sclerosing cholangitis. ACG Case Rep J. 2018:5:e54.

57. Lindor KD, Kowdley KV, Harrison ME. ACG Clinical Guideline: Primary sclerosing cholangitis. Am J Gastroenterol. 2015;110(5):646-659.

58. Bjornsson E, Lindqvist-Ottosson J, Asztely M et al. Dominant strictures in patients with primary sclerosing cholangitis. Am J Gastroenterol. 2004;99:502-508.

59. Tischendorf JJ, Kruger M, Trautwein C et al. Cholangioscopic characterization of dominant bile duct stenoses in patients with primary sclerosing cholangitis . Endoscopy. 2006;38:665–669.

60. Awadallah NS , Chen YK , Piraka C et al. Is there a role for cholangioscopy in patients with primary sclerosing cholangitis? Am J Gastroenterol. 2006;101:284–291.

61. Bangarulingam SY, Gossard AA, Petersen BT et al. Complications of endoscopic retrograde cholangiopancreatography in primary sclerosing cholangitis . Am J Gastroenterol. 2009;104:855-860.

62. Kulkarni C, Cholankeril G, Fardeen T, et al. Statin use is associated with protection against acute cholangitis in patients with primary sclerosing cholangitis: a multicenter retrospective cohort study. Clin Transl Gastroenterol. 2025 Apr 1;16(4):e00816.

63. Stokkeland K, Höijer J, Bottai M, et al. Statin use is associated with improved outcomes of patients with primary sclerosing cholangitis. Clin Gastroenterol Hepatol. 2019;17(9):1860-1866.

64. Baluyut AR, Sherman S, Lehman GA et al. Impact of endoscopic therapy on the survival of patients with primary sclerosing cholangitis. Gastrointest Endosc. 2001; 53:308–312.

65. Hammel P, Couvelard A, O'Toole D, et al. Regression of liver fibrosis after biliary drainage in patients with chronic pancreatitis and stenosis of the common bile duct. N Engl J Med. 2001; 344:418-423.

66. Rudolph G, Gotthardt D, Kloters-Plachky P, et al. Influence of dominant bile duct stenoses and biliary infections on outcome in primary sclerosing cholangitis. J Hepatol. 2009;51: 149-155.

67. Simkin P, Primary sclerosing cholangitis. Case study, Radiopaedia.org. Accessed 13 Jul 2025. https://doi.org/10.53347/rID-33367.

68. Soetikno RM, Lin OS, Heidenreich PA et al. Increased risk of colorectal neoplasia in patients with primary sclerosing cholangitis and ulcerative colitis: A meta-analysis . Gastrointest Endosc. 2002;56: 48–54.

69. Gonzalez RS. Primary sclerosing cholangitis. PathologyOutlines.com website. https://www.pathologyoutlines.com/topic/liverpsc.html. Accessed 13 July 2025

70. Gaillard F. Gallbladder polyp. Case study, Radiopaedia.org. Accessed 13 Jul 2025. https://doi.org/10.53347/rID-8151.

71. Eaton JE, Thackeray EW, Lindor KD . Likelihood of malignancy in gallbladder polyps and outcomes following cholecystectomy in primary sclerosing cholangitis. Am J Gastroenterol. 2012;107:431–439.

72. Razumilava N, Gores GJ, Lindor KD. Cancer surveillance in patients with primary sclerosing cholangitis. Hepatology. 2011;54:1842–1852.

73. Lewis JT, Talwalkar JA, Rosen CB, et al. Prevalence and risk factors for gallbladder neoplasia in patients with primary sclerosing cholangitis: Evidence for a metaplasia-dysplasia-carcinoma sequence. Am J Surg Pathol. 2007;31:907–913.

74. Shindoh J, de Aretxabala X, Aloia TA, et al. Tumor location is a strong predictor of tumor progression and survival in T2 gallbladder cancer: An international multicenter study. Ann Surg. 2015; 261:733.

75. Jophlin LL, Singal AK, Bataller R, et al. ACG Clinical Guideline: Alcohol-associated liver disease. Am J Gastroenterol. 2024;119(1):30–54.

76. Askgaard G, Kjaer MS, Tolstrup JS. Opportunities to prevent alcoholic liver cirrhosis in high-risk populations: A systematic review with meta-analysis. Am J Gastroenterol. 2019;114(2):221–32.

77. Babor TF, Higgins-Biddle JC, Saunders JB, Monteiro MG. AUDIT. The Alcohol Use Disorder Identification Test: Guidelines for Use in Primary Care, Second Edition. Geneva, Switzerland: World Health Organization; 2001.

78. Bataller R, Arab JP, Shah VH. Alcohol-associated hepatitis. N Engl J Med. 2022;387(26):2436–48.

79. Chen CM, Yoon Y-H. Liver Cirrhosis Mortality in the United States: National, State, and Regional Trends, 2000–2019. Sterling, VA: National Institutes of Health; 2022.

80. Singal AK, Arora S, Wong RJ, et al. Increasing burden of acute-on-chronic liver failure among alcohol-associated liver disease in the young population in the United States. Am J Gastroenterol. 2020;115(1):88–95.

81. Pollard MS, Tucker JS, Green HD Jr. Changes in adult alcohol use and consequences during the COVID-19 pandemic in the US. JAMA Netw Open. 2020;3(9):e2022942.

82. Yeo YH, He X, Ting PS, et al. Evaluation of trends in alcohol use disorder-related mortality in the US before and during the COVID-19 pandemic. JAMA Netw Open. 2022;5:e2210259.

83. Viel G, Boscolo-Berto R, Cecchetto G, et al. Phosphatidylethanol in blood as a marker of chronic alcohol use: A systematic review and meta analysis. Int J Mol Sci. 2012;13(11):14788–812.

84. Rogal S, Youk A, Zhang H, et al. Impact of alcohol use disorder treatment on clinical outcomes among patients with cirrhosis. Hepatology. 2020;71(6):2080–92.

85. Vannier AGL, Shay JES, Fomin V, et al. Incidence and progression of alcohol-associated liver disease after medical therapy for alcohol use disorder. JAMA Netw Open. 2022;5:e2213014.

86. Jophlin LL, Singal AK, Shah VH. Alcohol-associated liver disease. Am J Gastroenterol. 2025;120:495-499.

87. Holbeck M, DeVries HS, Singal AK. Integrated multidisciplinary management of alcohol-associated liver disease. J Clin Transl Hepatol. 2023;11(6):1404–12.

88. Singal AK, Wong RJ, Dasarathy S, et al. ACG Clinical Guideline: Malnutrition and nutritional recommendations in liver disease. Am J Gastroenterol. 2025;120(5):950-972.

89. Hart CL, Morrison DS, Batty GD, et al. Effect of body mass index and alcohol consumption on liver disease: Analysis of data from two prospective cohort studies. BMJ. 2010;340:c1240.

90. Marti-Aguado D, Calleja JL, Vilar-Gomez E, et al. Low-to-moderate alcohol consumption is associated with increased fibrosis in individuals with metabolic dysfunction-associated steatotic liver disease. J Hepatol. 2024;81(6):930-940.

91. Loomba R, Yang HI, Su J, et al. Obesity and alcohol synergize to increase the risk of incident hepatocellular carcinoma in men. Clin Gastroenterol Hepatol. 2010;8(10):891–898, 898.e1-2.

92. Frezza M, di Padova C, Pozzato G, et al. High blood alcohol levels in women. The role of decreased gastric alcohol dehydrogenase activity and first-pass metabolism. N Engl J Med. 1990;322(2):95–9.

93. Beaudoin JJ, Long N, Liangpunsakul S, et al. An exploratory genomewide analysis of genetic risk for alcoholic hepatitis. Scand J Gastroenterol. 2017;52(11):1263–9.

94. Atkinson SR, Way MJ, McQuillin A, et al. Homozygosity for rs738409:G in PNPLA3 is associated with increased mortality following an episode of severe alcoholic hepatitis. J Hepatol. 2017;67(1):120–7.

95. Kim HP, Jiang Y, Farrell TM, et al. Roux-en-Y gastric bypass is associated with increased hazard for de novo alcohol-related complications and liver disease. J Clin Gastroenterol. 2022;56(2):181–5.

96. Klatsky AL, Armstrong MA. Alcohol, smoking, coffee, and cirrhosis. Am J Epidemiol. 1992;136(10):1248–57.

97. Dam MK, Flensborg-Madsen T, Eliasen M, et al. Smoking and risk of liver cirrhosis: A population-based cohort study. Scand J Gastroenterol. 2013;48(5):585–91.

98. Mendenhall C, Roselle GA, Gartside P, et al. Relationship of protein calorie malnutrition to alcoholic liver disease: A reexamination of data from two Veterans Administration cooperative studies. Alcohol Clin Exp Res. 1995;19(3):635–41.

99. Eslamparast T, Montano-Loza AJ, Raman M, et al. Sarcopenic obesity in cirrhosis-the confluence of 2 prognostic titans. Liver Int. 2018;38(10):1706–17.

100. McClain CJ, Barve SS, Barve A, Marsano L. Alcoholic liver disease and malnutrition. Alcohol Clin Exp Res. 2011;35(5):815-20.

101. Spiegel B and Karsan HA. *Acing the Hepatology Questions on the GI Board Exam: The Ultimate Crunch-Time Resource*. Thorofare, NJ: SLACK Incorporated; 2012.

102. Maddrey WC, Boitnott JK, Bedine MS, et al. Corticosteroid therapy of alcoholic hepatitis. Gastroenterology. 1978;75(2):193–9.

103. Gholam PM. Prognosis and prognostic scoring models for alcoholic liver disease and acute alcoholic hepatitis. Clin Liver Dis. 2016;20(3):491–7.

104. Mathurin P, O'Grady J, Carithers RL, et al. Corticosteroids improve short-term survival in patients with severe alcoholic hepatitis: Metaanalysis of individual patient data. Gut. 2011;60(2):255–60.

105. Garcia-Saenz-de-Sicilia M, Duvoor C, Altamirano J, et al. A day-4 Lille model predicts response to corticosteroids and mortality in severe alcoholic hepatitis. Am J Gastroenterol. 2017;112(2):306–15.

106. Thursz MR, Richardson P, Allison M, et al. Prednisolone or pentoxifylline for alcoholic hepatitis. N Engl J Med. 2015;372(17): 1619–28.

107. Louvet A, Diaz E, Dharancy S, et al. Early switch to pentoxifylline in patients with severe alcoholic hepatitis is inefficient in non-responders to corticosteroids. J Hepatol. 2008;48(3):465–70.

108. Louvet A, Labreuche J, Dao T, et al. Effect of prophylactic antibiotics on mortality in severe alcohol-related hepatitis: A randomized clinical trial. JAMA. 2023; 329(18):1558–1566.

109. Singh S, Murad MH, Chandar AK, et al. Comparative effectiveness of pharmacological interventions for severe alcoholic hepatitis: A systematic review and network meta-analysis. Gastroenterology. 2015;149(4):958–970.

110. Mathurin P, Moreno C, Samuel D, et al. Early liver transplantation for severe alcoholic hepatitis. N Engl J Med. 2011;365(19):1790–800.

111. Musto JA, Palmer G, Nemer S, et al. Early liver transplant for alcohol-associated liver disease has excellent survival but higher rates of harmful alcohol use. Clin Gastroenterol Hepatol. 2024;22(8):1646-1656.

112. Kwo PY, Cohen SM, Lim JK. ACG Clinical Guideline: Evaluation of Abnormal Liver Chemistries. Am J Gastroenterol. 2017; 112:18–35.

113. Lee TH, Kim WR, Benson JT, et al. Serum aminotransferase activity and mortality risk in a United States community. Hepatology. 2008; 47:880–887.

114. Ruhl CE, Everhart JE. Elevated serum alanine aminotransferase and gamma-glutamyltransferase and mortality in the United States population. Gastroenterology. 2009; 136 (477-85): e11.

115. Sterling RK, Lissen E, Clumeck N, et al. Development of a simple noninvasive index to predict significant fibrosis in patients with HIV/HCV coinfection. Hepatology. 2006;43(6):1317-1325.

116. Kanwal F, Neuschwander-Tetri BA, Loomba R, et al. Metabolic dysfunction-associated steatotic liver disease: Update and impact of new nomenclature on the American Association for the Study of Liver Diseases practice guidance on nonalcoholic fatty liver disease. Hepatology. 2024;79(5):1212-1219.

117. European Association for the Study of the Liver (EASL); European Association for the Study of Diabetes (EASD); European Association for the Study of Obesity (EASO). EASL-EASD-EASO Clinical Practice Guidelines on the management of metabolic

dysfunction-associated steatotic liver disease (MASLD). J Hepatol. 2024;81(3):492-542.

118. Promrat K, Kleiner DE, Niemeier HM, et al. Randomized controlled trial testing the effects of weight loss on nonalcoholic steatohepatitis. Hepatology. 2010;51(1):121-129.

119. Kaplan MM. Alkaline phosphatase . N Engl J Med. 1972;286:200–202.

120. Shingina A, Mukhtar N, Wakim-Fleming J, Alqahtani S, Wong RJ, Limketkai BN, Larson AM, Grant L. Acute liver failure guidelines. Am J Gastroenterol. 2023; 118(7):1128-1153.

121. Harrison PM, Keays R, Bray GP, et al. Improved outcome of paracetamol-induced fulminant hepatic failure by late administration of acetylcysteine. Lancet. 1990; 335(8705):1572–1573.

122. Rumack BH, Matthew H. Acetaminophen poisoning and toxicity. Pediatrics. 1975;55(6):871-876.

123. Buckley NA, Whyte IM, O'Connell DL, et al. Activated charcoal reduces the need for N-acetylcysteine treatment after acetaminophen (paracetamol) overdose. J Toxicol Clin Toxicol. 1999;37(6):753–757.

124. O'Grady J, Alexander G, Hayllar K, Williams R. Early indicators of prognosis in fulminant hepatic failure. Gastroenterology. 1989; 97 (2): 439–445.

125. McPhail MJW, Farne H, Senvar N, et al. Ability of King's College criteria and model for end-stage liver disease scores to predict mortality of patients with acute liver failure: A meta-analysis. Clin Gastroenterol Hepatol. 2016;14(4):516–25.

126. Walayat S, Shoaib H, Asghar M, et al. Role of N-acetylcysteine in nonacetaminophen-related acute liver failure: An updated meta-analysis and systematic review. Ann Gastroenterol. 2021;34(2):235–240.

127. Stravitz RT, Ellerbe C, Durkalski V, et al. Bleeding complications in acute liver failure. Hepatology. 2018;67(5):1931–1942.

128. Stravitz RT, Lisman T, Luketic VA, et al. Minimal effects of acute liver injury/acute liver failure on hemostasis as assessed by thromboelastography. J Hepatol. 2012;56(1):129–36.

129. Chalasani NP, Maddur H, Russo MW, Wong RJ, Reddy KR. ACG Clinical Guideline: Diagnosis and management of idiosyncratic drug-induced liver injury. Am J Gastroenterol. 2021;116(5):878-898.

130. Temple R. Hy's law: Predicting serious hepatotoxicity. Pharmacoepidemiol Drug Saf. 2006;15(4):241–3.

131. Peeraphatdit TB, Wang J, Odenwald MA, et al. Hepatotoxicity from immune checkpoint inhibitors: A systematic review and management recommendation. Hepatology. 2020;72(1):315–29.

132. Bajaj JS, O'Leary JG, Lai JC, et al. Acute-on-chronic liver failure clinical guidelines. Am J Gastroenterol. 2022;117:225-252.

133. Bajaj JS, Moreau R, Kamath PS, et al. Acute-on-chronic liver failure: Getting ready for prime-time. Hepatology. 2018;68(4):1621–32.

134. Bajaj JS, O'Leary JG, Reddy KR, Wong F, Biggins SW, Patton H, et al. Survival in infection-related acute-on-chronic liver failure is defined by extrahepatic organ failures. Hepatology. 2014;60(1):250–256.

135. European Association for the Study of the Liver. EASL Clinical Practice Guidelines on acute-on-chronic liver failure. J Hepatol. 2023;79(2):461-491.

136. Sarin SK, Choudhury A, Sharma MK, et al. Acute-on-chronic liver failure: Consensus recommendations of the Asian Pacific association for the study of the liver (APASL): An update. Hepatol Int. 2019;13:353–90.

137. Seymour CW, Gesten F, Prescott HC, et al. Time to treatment and mortality during mandated emergency care for sepsis. N Engl J Med. 2017;376:2235–44.

138. Sort P, Navasa M, Arroyo V, et al. Effect of intravenous albumin on renal impairment and mortality in patients with cirrhosis and spontaneous bacterial peritonitis. N Engl J Med. 1999;341:403–9.

139. O'Leary JG, Reddy KR, Garcia-Tsao G, et al. NACSELD acute-on-chronic liver failure (NACSELD-ACLF) score predicts 30-day survival in hospitalized patients with cirrhosis. Hepatology. 2018; 67: 2367-2374.

140. Angeli P, Garcia-Tsao G, Nadim MK, Parikh CR. News in pathophysiology, definition and classification of hepatorenal syndrome: A step beyond the International Club of Ascites (ICA) consensus document. J Hepatol. 2019 Oct;71(4):811-822.

141. Frenette C, Mendiratta-Lalla M, Salgia R, Wong RJ, Sauer BG, Pillai A. ACG Clinical Guideline: Focal liver lesions. Am J Gastroenterol. 2024;119:1235-1271.

142. Orcutt ST, Kobayashi K, Sultenfuss M, et al. Portal vein embolization as an oncosurgical strategy prior to major hepatic resection: Anatomic, surgical, and technical considerations. Front Surg. 2016;3:14.

143. Elbanna KY, Kielar AZ. Computed tomography versus magnetic resonance imaging for hepatic lesion characterization/diagnosis. Clin Liver Dis (Hoboken). 2021;17(3):159–64.

144. Di Muzio B, Hepatic hemangiomas. Case study, Radiopaedia.org. Accessed 13 Jul 2025. https://doi.org/10.53347/rID-20956.

145. Niknejad M, Focal nodular hyperplasia (FNH). Case study, Radiopaedia.org. Accessed13 Jul 2025. https://doi.org/10.53347/rID-64211.

146. D'Onofrio M, Rozzanigo U, Masinielli BM, et al. Hypoechoic focal liver lesions: characterization with contrast enhanced ultrasonography. J Clin Ultrasound. 2005 May;33(4):164-72.

147. Singal AG, Llovet JM, Yarchoan M, et al. AASLD practice guidance on prevention, diagnosis, and treatment of hepatocellular carcinoma. Hepatology. 2023;78(6):1922–65.

148. European Association for the Study of the Liver. EASL Clinical Practice Guidelines on the management of hepatocellular carcinoma. J Hepatol. 2025;82(2):315-374.

149. Chernyak V, Fowler KJ, Kamaya A, et al. Liver Imaging Reporting and Data System (LI-RADS) version 2018: Imaging of hepatocellular carcinoma in at-risk patients. Radiology. 2018;289(3):816–830.

150. Tang A, Bashir MR, Corwin MT, Cruite I, Dietrich CF, et al. ; LI-RADS Evidence Working Group. Evidence supporting LI-RADS major features for CT- and MR imaging-based diagnosis of hepatocellular carcinoma: A systematic review. Radiology. 2018;286:29–48.

151. Singal AG, et al. Comparison of a multitarget blood test to ultrasound and alpha-fetoprotein for hepatocellular carcinoma surveillance: Results of a network meta-analysis. Hepatol Commun. 2022;6(10):2925–2936.

152. Nault JC, Couchy G, Balabaud C, et al. Molecular classification of hepatocellular adenoma associates with risk factors, bleeding, and malignant transformation. Gastroenterology. 2017;152(4):880–894.

153. Farges O, Ferreira N, Dokmak S, et al. Changing trends in malignant transformation of hepatocellular adenoma. Gut. 2011;60(1):85–89.

154. Tran TT, Ahn J, Reau NS. ACG Clinical Guideline: Liver Disease and Pregnancy. Am J Gastroenterol. 2016;111(2):176-194.

155. Robson SC, Mutch E, Boys RJ et al. Apparent liver blood flow during pregnancy: a serial study using indocyanine green clearance. Br J Obstet Gynaecol. 1990;97:720–3.

156. Elinav E, Ben-Dov IZ, Shapira Y et al. Acute hepatitis A infection in pregnancy is associated with high rates of gestational complications and preterm labor. Gastroenterology. 2006;130:129-134.

157. Watson JC, Fleming DW, Borella AJ, et al. Vertical transmission of hepatitis A resulting in an outbreak in a neonatal intensive care unit. J Infect Dis. 1993;167: 567–571.

158. European Association for the Study of the Liver. EASL Clinical Practice Guidelines on the management of hepatitis B virus infection. J Hepatol. 2025;83(2):502-583.

159. Han G-R, Cao M-K, Zhao W et al. A prospective and open label study for the efficacy and safety of telbivudine in pregnancy for the prevention of perinatal transmission of hepatitis B virus infection. J Hepatology. 2011;55:1215–1221.

160. Benova L, Mohamoud YA, Calvert C, Abu-Raddad LJ. Vertical transmission of hepatitis C virus: systematic review and meta-analysis. Clin Infect Dis. 2014;15;59(6):765-73.

161. Cottrell EB, Chou R, Wasson N, et al. Reducing risk for mother-to-infant transmission of hepatitis C virus: a systematic review for the U.S. Preventive Services Task Force. Ann Intern Med. 2013; 158:109-113.

162. Patra S, Kumar A, Trivedi SS, et al. Maternal and fetal outcomes in pregnant women with acute hepatitis E virus infection. Ann Intern Med. 2007;147:28–33.

163. Levitsky J, Duddempudi AT, Lakeman FD, et al. Detection and diagnosis of herpes simplex virus infection in adults with acute liver failure. Liver Transpl. 2008;14:1498–504.

164. Norvell JP, Blei AT, Jovanovic BD, Levitsky J. Herpes simplex virus hepatitis: an analysis of the published literature and institutional cases. Liver Transpl. 2007;13(10):1428-34.

165. Olson, KM, Keim, LM, Tyson, T, et al. Hepatic microabscesses: A unique presentation of herpes simplex virus hepatitis. ACG Case Reports Journal 8(12): e00697, December 2021.

166. Hidaka M, Takatsuki M, Soyama A, et al. Living donor liver transplantation from a donor previously treated with interferon for hepatitis C virus: A case report. J Med Case Rep. 2011 Jul 3;5:276.

167. Goodwin TM . Hyperemesis gravidarum. Clin Obstet Gynecol. 2008;35:40-17.

168. Bottomley C, Bourne T. Management strategies for hyperemesis. Best practice & research. Clin Obstet Gynecol. 2009; 23:549-564.

169. Williamson C, Hems LM, Goulis DG et al. Clinical outcome in a series of cases of obstetric cholestasis identified via a patient support group. BJOG 2004;111:676.

170. Bacq Y, Sentilhes L, Reyes HB et al. Efficacy of ursodeoxycholic acid in treating intrahepatic cholestasis of pregnancy: A meta-analysis. Gastroenterology. 2012;143:1492.

171. Knight M, Nelson-Peircy C, Kurinczuk JJ, et al. A prospective national study of acute fatty liver of pregnancy in the UK. Gut. 2008;57(7):951-956.

172. Ockner SA, Brunt EM, Cohn SM et al. Fulminant hepatic failure caused by acute fatty liver of pregnancy treated by orthotopic liver transplantation. Hepatology. 1990;11:59–64.

173. Goel A, Ramakrishna B, Zachariah U, et al. How accurate are the Swansea criteria to diagnose acute fatty liver of pregnancy in predicting hepatic microvesicular steatosis? Gut. 2011;60:138–9.

174. Tandra S, Yeh MM, Brunt EM, et al. Presence and significance of microvesicular steatosis in nonalcoholic fatty liver disease. J Hepatol. 2011 Sep;55(3):654-659.

175. Vigil-De Gracia P, Ortega-Paz L. Pre-eclampsia/eclampsia and hepatic rupture. Int J Gynaecol Obstet. 2012;118:186-189.

176. Churchill D, Duley L, Thornton JG, Moussa M, Ali HS, Walker KF. Interventionist versus expectant care for severe pre-eclampsia between 24 and 34 weeks' gestation. Cochrane Database Syst Rev. 2018;10(10):CD003106.

177. Koopmans CM, Bijlenga D, Groen H et al. Induction of labour versus expectant monitoring for gestational hypertension or mild pre-eclampsia aft er 36 weeks' gestation (HYPITAT): A multicentre, open-label randomised controlled trial . Lancet. 2009;374:979–88.

178. Mikolajczyk AE, Renz J, Diaz G, Alpert L, Hart J, Te HS. Massive hepatic infarction caused by HELLP Syndrome. ACG Case Rep J. 2017;4:e81.

179. Anwar AD, Nugrahani AD, Amaluna Zahra T, et al. How to Differentiate Acute Fatty Liver in Pregnancy (AFLP) with Hemolysis, Elevated Liver Enzymes, and Low Platelets (HELLP) Syndrome in Resource-Limited Settings? - The Importance of Swansea Criteria. Eur J Obstet Gynecol Reprod Biol X. 2023 Jan 10;17:100176.

180. Kowdley KV, Brown KE, Ahn J, Sundaram V. ACG Clinical Guideline: Hereditary Hemochromatosis. Am J Gastroenterol. 2019;114:1202-1218.

181. Adams PC, Reboussin DM, Press RD, et al. Biological variability of transferrin saturation and unsaturated iron-binding capacity. Am J Med. 2007;120(11):999.e1-7.

182. Morrison ED, Brandhagen DJ, Phatak PD, et al. Serum ferritin level predicts advanced hepatic fibrosis among U.S. patients with phenotypic hemochromatosis. Ann Intern Med. 2003;138(8):627–633.

183. Strohmeyer G, Niederau C, Stremmel W. Survival and causes of death in hemochromatosis: Observations in 163 patients. AnnNYAcad Sci. 1988; 526:245–257.

184. Sarigianni M, Liakos A, Vlachaki E, et al. Accuracy of magnetic resonance imaging in diagnosis of liver iron overload: A systematic review and meta-analysis. Clin Gastroenterol Hepatol. 2015;13(1): 55–63.

185. Blumberg RS, Chopra S, Ibrahim R, et al. Primary hepatocellular carcinoma in idiopathic hemochromatosis after reversal of cirrhosis. Gastroenterology. 1988;95(5):1399–1402.

186. Simonetto DA, Singal AK, Garcia-Tsao G, Caldwell SH, Ahn J, Kamath PS. ACG Clinical Guideline: Disorders of the hepatic and mesenteric circulation. Am J Gastroenterol. 2020;115(1):18-40.

187. Plessier A, Darwish-Murad S, Hernandez-Guerra M, et al. Acute portal vein thrombosis unrelated to cirrhosis: A prospective multicenter follow-up study. Hepatology. 2010;51:210–8.

188. Englesbe MJ, Kubus J, Muhammad W, et al. Portal vein thrombosis and survival in patients with cirrhosis. Liver Transpl. 2010;16:83–90.

189. Rizk M, Budd-Chiari syndrome. Case study, Radiopaedia.org. Accessed 13 Jul 2025. https://doi.org/10.53347/rID-171826.

190. PatelRK, LeaNC, HeneghanMA, etal. Prevalence of the activating JAK2 tyrosine kinase mutation V617F in the Budd-Chiari syndrome. Gastroenterology 2006;130:2031–8.

Image Credits

Images used from the ACG Guidelines are reproduced in this book under the permission of the American College of Gastroenterology.

The authors retain the rights to all mnemonics presented in the series.

Figure 1.2 Image reproduced from Saleh H et al, ACG Case Rep J. 2024.[14]
Figure 1.5 *CBD stones.jpg* by Samir CC BY-SA 3.0.
Figure 1.6 *MRCP Pankreas divisum.jpg* by Hellerhoff CC BY-SA 3.0
Figure 1.8 Image courtesy of Praveen Jah, Radiopaedia.org, rID 16287
Figure 1.9 Image courtesy of Erik Ranschaert, Radiopaedia.org, rID 11060
Figures 1.10 and 1.11 are reproduced from Oh HC, et al, Am J Gastroenterol. 2008[36]
Figure 1.12 Image reproduced Malekzadeh S al[37] under an open access license.
Figure 2.1 *ERCP cholangioca.jpg* by Samir CC BY-SA 4.0.
Figure 2.2 Image reproduced from Coté et al[47] under an open access license.
Figure 2.3 Image reproduced from CastañoLlano[54] under an open access license.
Figure 2.4 Image reproduced from Sundaram S et al, ACG Case Rep J. 2018.[56]
Figure 2.5 Image courtesy of Paul Simkin, Radiopaedia.org, rID 33367
Figure 2.6 Image courtesy of Raul S. Gonzalez, M.D., and PathologyOutlines.com.
Figure 2.7 Image courtesy of Frank Gaillard, Radiopaedia.org, rID 8151.
Figure 3.1 Image courtesy of Romil Saxena, MD.
Figure 3.2 Used with permission from McClain CJ, Alcohol Clin Exp Res. 2011.[100]
Figure 3.8 *Kayser-Fleisher_ring.jpg* by Filip em CC BY-SA 3.0
Figure 3.12 Case courtesy of Bruno Di Muzio, Radiopaedia.org, rID: 20956.
Figure 3.13 Case courtesy of Mohammad Taghi Niknejad , Radiopaedia.org, rID: 64211.
Figure 3.14 Images courtesy of Anjana Pillai, MD, FACG.
Figure 3.15 Used with permission from Wiley Periodicals, Inc., A Wiley Company. D'Onofrio M et al. J Clin Ultrasound. 2005.[146]
Figure 3.16 Used with permission by the Radiological Society of North America, Inc. Chernyak V et al, Radiology. 2018.[149]
Figure 3.18 Image reproduced from Olson KM et al, ACG Case Rep J. 2021.[165]
Figure 3.19 Image reproduced from Hidaka M et al[166] under an open access license.
Figure 3.20 Used with permission from European Association for the Study of the Liver, Tandra S et al, J Hepatol. 2011[174]
Figures 3.21 and 3.22 are reproduced from Mikolajczyk AE, et al, ACG Case Rep J. 2017.[178]
Figure 3.25 Image courtesy of Mina Sameh Rizk, Radiopaedia.org, rID: 171826.

Abbreviations

ACG, American College of Gastroenterology
ACLF, acute-on-chronic liver failure
AFLP, acute fatty liver of pregnancy
AH, alcohol-associated hepatitis
AIH, autoimmune hepatitis
AJG, *The American Journal of Gastroenterology*
AKI, acute kidney infection
ALD, alcohol-associated liver disease
ALF, acute liver failure
ALP, alkaline phosphatase
ALT, alanne aminotransferase
ANA, Antinuclear Antibody
ANC, acute necrotic collection
AP, acute pancreatitis
ASMA, anti-smooth muscle antibody
AST, aspartate aminotransferase
AUD, alcohol use disorder
BCS, Budd-Chiari Syndrome
BMI, body mass index
BP, blood pressure
BUN, blood urea nitrogen
CBD, common bile duct
CCA, cholangiocarcinoma
CT, computed tomography
Cr, creatinine
DOAC, direct oral anticoagulant
ED, emergency department
EPI, exocrine pancreatic insufficiency
ERCP, endoscopic retrograde cholangiopancreatography
EUS, endoscopic ultrasound
FISH, fluorescence in situ hybridization
FNA, fine needle aspiration
FNB, fine needle biopsy
GGT, gamma-glutamyl transferase
GI, gastrointestinal
HAV, hepatitis A virus

HCV, hepatitis C virus
HEV, hepatitis E virus
HCC, hepatocellular carcinoma
HCT, hematocrit
HH, hereditary hemochromatosis
HR, heart rate
HRS, hepatorenal syndrome
HSV, herpes simplex virus
HTG, hypertriglyceridemiac
IBD, inflammatory bowel disease
ICP, intracranial pressure
ICU, intensive care unit
Ig, Immunoglobulin
INR, international normalized ratio
IV, intravenous
LR, lactated Ringer's
LUQ, left upper quadrant
MASLD, metabolic dysfunction-associated steatotic liver disease
MELD, Model for End-Stage Liver Disease
MRCP, magnetic resonance cholangiopancreatography
MRI, magnetic resonance imaging
NPO, nil per os; nothing by mouth
NG, nasogastric
NJ, nasojejunal
NS, normal saline
NSAID, non-steroidal anti-inflammatory drugs
PCA, patient controlled analgesia
PCR, polymerase chain reaction
PMN, polymorphonuclear leukocyte
PSC, primary sclerosing cholangitis
PVT, portal vein thrombosis
RCT, randomized controlled trial
RR, respiratory rate
RUQ, right upper quadrant
SCA, serous cystadenoma
SIRS, Systemic Inflammatory Response Syndrome
TACE, transarterial chemoembolization

TARE, transarterial radioembolization
TG, triglyceride
TPIAT, total pancreatectomy with islet autotransplantation
TSAT, transferrin saturation
UDCA, ursodeoxycholic acid
ULN, upper limit of normal
WBC, white blood cell

www.ingramcontent.com/pod-product-compliance
Lightning Source LLC
LaVergne TN
LVHW050928210926
848482LV00013B/563

* 9 7 9 8 2 1 8 8 2 4 8 6 0 *